The Royal Marsden Hospital Handbook
of Wound Management in Cancer Care

The Royal Marsden Hospital Handbook of Wound Management in Cancer Care

Wayne Naylor

BSC, DIP NURSING, RN, ONC CERT
Wound Management Research Nurse
Directorate of Nursing, Rehabilitation and Quality Assurance
The Royal Marsden Hospital

Diane Laverty

BSC, RGN, ONC CERT
Clinical Nurse Specialist Palliative Care
Directorate of Nursing, Rehabilitation and Quality Assurance
The Royal Marsden Hospital

Jane Mallett

PHD, MSC, BSC, RGN
Nursing and Rehabilitation Research and Development Manager
Directorate of Nursing, Rehabilitation and Quality Assurance
The Royal Marsden Hospital

Blackwell Science

Contents

Contents

Contributors

Amanda Baxter BSc, RN, RMN (Onc Cert)
Clinical Nurse Specialist Pelvic Care (Chapter 3)

Sarah Hart MSc, BSc, RN, FETC, Onc Cert
Clinical Nurse Specialist Infection Control and Radiation Protection (Chapter 3)

Diane Laverty BSc, RN, Onc Cert
Clinical Nurse Specialist Palliative Care (Chapters 2, 3, 4 and 5)

Jane Mallett PhD, MSc, BSc, RN
Nursing and Rehabilitation Research and Development Manager (Chapter 4)

Wayne Naylor BSc, Dip Nursing, RN, Onc Cert
Wound Management Research Nurse (Chapters 1, 2, 3, 4 and 5)

Caroline Soady BSc, RN
Clinical Nurse Specialist Head, Neck and Thyroid (Chapters 4 and 5)

Miriam Wood BSc, RN, Onc Cert
Informatics Project Nurse (Chapter 2)

(All at The Royal Marsden Hospital)

PREVIOUS CONTRIBUTORS (to The Royal Marsden Hospital wound management guidelines)
Jane Mulholland, formerly Principal Pharmacist, The Royal Marsden Hospital

Deborah Fenlon, Lecturer, Centre for Cancer and Palliative Care Studies

Frances Fuller, formerly Clinical Nurse Specialist Lung Cancer, The Royal Marsden Hospital

Foreword

I have a confession to make! I can now openly admit that early in my clinical career as a Registered Nurse my knowledge of wound management was woefully inadequate. I clearly remember being aware of my limitations in this area at that time. During those first years of my professional practice I gradually cobbled together a somewhat haphazard knowledge base from study days, reading articles and pestering the Ward Sister to help me. I think that eventually I developed a reasonable level of clinical expertise in wound management. However, wound management is a core nursing skill and all patients should be afforded up-to-date and competent nursing care of their wounds. An evidence-based resource like *The Royal Marsden Hospital Handbook of Wound Management in Cancer Care* would have been enormously useful to me and would have improved the care I offered to my patients. With this in mind, I feel that this work will be welcomed by nurses and other members of the multidisciplinary team who need to find up-to-date and accurate information on wound management quickly and easily.

This Handbook has been published in 2001, a year marking the 150th anniversary of The Royal Marsden Hospital, which opened in 1851 as the first specialist cancer hospital in the world. The sharing of good nursing practice is recognised as an important part of our work and it is certainly a core commitment for the future. This Handbook is an excellent example of that commitment.

My personal experience as a clinical nurse certainly influenced my decision to support the work that produced this Handbook and, in particular, to seek funding from our most generous supporters at The Royal Marsden to complete this project. I would like to take this opportunity to thank the Editors, Wayne Naylor, Diane Laverty and Jane Mallett, for their tenacity, persistence and hard work.

Dickon Weir-Hughes
Chief Nurse and Director of Quality Assurance
The Royal Marsden Hospital (London & Surrey)

Acknowledgements

Dr Karen Broadley, Consultant, Palliative Medicine, The Royal Marsden Hospital

Mercel Ball, Senior Staff Nurse, Weston Ward, The Royal Marsden Hospital

Tracey Cricket, Radiographer, The Royal Marsden Hospital

Dr Janet Hardy, Consultant, Palliative Care, The Royal Marsden Hospital

Rachel Mead, Sister, Ellis Ward, The Royal Marsden Hospital

Sandy Miller, Senior Staff Nurse Outpatient Department, The Royal Marsden Hospital

Diane O'Connell, formerly Sister, Outpatient Department, The Royal Marsden Hospital

Vina Patel, Senior Staff Nurse, Outpatient Department, The Royal Marsden Hospital

Karen Summerville, formerly Clinical Nurse Specialist, The Royal Marsden Hospital

Ann and Tony Rose, The Monte Challenge

Dr Tamara Fishman, Podiatric Wound Consultant, Primary Foot Care Center Inc, Florida, USA

Sara Allen, Sales Representative, Johnson & Johnson Medical, Berkshire, UK

The Royal Marsden Hospital League of Friends (London) has generously supported the post of Wound Management Research Nurse. This has enabled the development of this Handbook along with many other wound management initiatives within The Royal Marsden Hospital. The Editors, on behalf of The Royal Marsden Hospital, would like to thank the League of Friends for their significant contribution to ensuring best practice in the care of oncology patients with chronic and/or complex wounds.

The Editors would like to thank all of those patients and carers who kindly gave permission for us to take and use many of the photographs that illustrate this book. We would also like to thank the two reviewers, Dr Steve Thomas and Ms Judith Coleman, for their insightful and very useful comments, and the Medical Photography Departments at the Chelsea and Sutton sites of the hospital for their hard work in preparing slides and photographs for use in this book.

Introduction

AIM

The Royal Marsden Hospital Handbook of Wound Management in Cancer Care has been developed to promote evidence-based, cost-effective management of wounds.

BACKGROUND

The Handbook has been developed from published research findings and professional opinion papers as well as the accumulated experience of an interdisciplinary team, including nurses, pharmacists and doctors with expertise in wound care, and the Wound Management Group at The Royal Marsden Hospital. The Handbook has been developed for use by both community and hospital-based nurses, particularly those providing care for oncology patients with complex and/or chronic wounds. However, it is anticipated that the Handbook will also be a useful resource for other health care professionals and pharmacists who require guidance and information on wound management. Health care professionals working in clinical areas other than oncology will also be able to utilise the Handbook when wounds require skilled management. While this book is intended to assist nursing practice and is based on the best available evidence, individual patient circumstances and professional judgement should be taken into account when planning patient care in order to provide a high quality and co-ordinated approach to wound management.

The Handbook provides a detailed outline of the management of specific wound symptoms that may appear either in isolation or in combination, including wound necrosis and infection. In addition, the handbook also incorporates the care of wounds that occur as a result of cancer or its treatments. This includes fungating wounds, acute skin reactions to radiotherapy, the management of graft versus host disease of the skin and plastic surgery wounds. To facilitate cost-effectiveness, particular wound care products are identified to manage different symptoms.

The Handbook has been designed to be used in conjunction with *The Royal Marsden Hospital Manual of Clinical Nursing Procedures* (Mallett & Dougherty 2000) and *Patient Group Directions* for nurse supply and administration of medicines developed within The Royal Marsden Hospital (Laverty *et al.* 1997, Mallett *et al.* 1997, Mallett & Dougherty 2000). Used together, these resources will ensure the highest quality holistic management for patients with simple or complex wounds (Mallett *et al.* 1999).

.

While this book provides detailed information on many different methods of wound management, health care professionals are reminded of the need to carry out patient care according to their level of competency and within their Scope of Practice (UKCC 1992). Finally, every effort has been made in the writing of this book to present accurate and up-to-date information from the best and most reliable sources. However, the result of managing patients' wounds depends upon a variety of factors not under the control of the authors. Therefore the authors do not assume responsibility for, nor make any warranty with respect to, the outcomes achieved from the information described therein

1   Physiology of Wound Healing

STRUCTURE OF THE SKIN AND THE NORMAL HEALING PROCESS

Introduction

Knowledge of wound healing physiology is not the sole domain of specialist practitioners, it is a basic area of understanding that all health care professionals involved in wound management need to have. By being aware of the phases that a wound progresses through during healing, and the factors that influence this process, the health care professional is able to maintain an effective and appropriate wound management strategy. This chapter looks at the structure and function of the skin, the normal healing process and factors that may have an influence on tissue repair.

Structure and function of the skin

The skin is one of the largest organs of the body. In the average adult the skin weighs about 5 kg and covers an area of around $2 m^2$ (Tortora & Grabowski 1996). While it is highly valued for its outward appearance, the physiological functions of the skin as a major body organ are often underestimated. It is a highly complex structure that performs a number of very important functions. The skin and its various appendages, hair, glands, nails and nerves, combine to form the integumentary system.

Skin is composed of two main layers, the epidermis and the dermis. Below the dermis is fatty tissue, known as the subcutaneous layer, which is attached to underlying muscle and bone (Collier 1996, Tortora & Grabowski 1996). Figure 1.1 is a diagrammatic representation of the skin and its structures.

The epidermis

The epidermis can be further divided into four or five layers depending on its location on the body (Fig. 1.1). The outer layer is the 'stratum corneum' and consists of dead cells (keratinocytes) filled with keratin. This layer is waterproof and provides protection from bacteria, heat and a number of chemicals (Tortora & Grabowski 1996). The stratum corneum is constantly replaced as cells slough

1

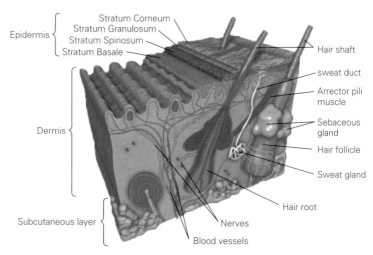

Fig. 1.1 Structure of the skin (© 1993–1995 SoftKey Multimedia Inc, a subsidiary of SoftKey International Inc, all rights reserved).

off through normal wear and tear: the whole layer is renewed approximately every 24 hours (Collier 1996).

In most other areas of the body, the second layer of the epidermis is the 'stratum granulosum'. The cells in this layer are also flattened and are in various stages of degeneration; however the cells are still active and contain granules of keratin (Ross *et al.* 1995).

The third layer is the 'stratum spinosum', which is several cells thick. This layer contains live cells that are tightly joined together by numerous processes on their cell membranes; the junctions connecting the cells are called desmosomes. Under a light microscope the cell processes look like spines and hence cells in this layer are commonly called prickle cells; they may also be referred to as squamous cells. The cells in this layer become flattened as they move upwards (Ross *et al.* 1995, Tortora & Grabowski 1996).

The final layer of the epidermis is the 'stratum basale' (also called the stratum germinativum). At this level there is a single layer of cuboidal cells that are multiplying and moving upwards to become part of the previously mentioned layers until they finally reach the stratum corneum and are shed. This layer also extends down to line the surface of hair follicles and sweat glands (Ross *et al.*

1995). When the epidermis is damaged it is the stratum basale that plays a vital role in the generation of new cells to repair the defect (Collier 1996).

In the soles of the feet and palms of the hand, there is an extra layer beneath the stratum corneum called the 'stratum lucidum'. This is a specialised layer only found in thick skin and contains dead, flattened cells filled with a substance called eleidin (Tortora & Grabowski 1996). It provides a cushioning effect to reduce surface impact.

Within the epidermis there are four cell types:

(1) *Keratinocytes* – these are the predominant cell of the epidermis (approximately 90%) and produce keratin.
(2) *Melanocytes* – these are pigment-producing cells found in the stratum basale, they extend projections between cells of the stratum spinosum and transfer granules of melanin to keratinocytes.
(3) *Langerhans cells* – these cells arise in the bone marrow and are involved in cell-mediated immune responses in the skin (including contact sensitivities such as allergic dermatitis).
(4) *Merkel cells* – also located in the stratum basale, these cells are closely associated with sensory nerve endings and are involved in touch sensation (Ross *et al.* 1995, Strete 1995, Tortora & Grabowski 1996).

When damage to the skin is only as deep as the epidermal layer, it is able to 'regenerate' itself from cells in the stratum basale, which divide and fill the defect with cells the same as those that were originally there. Therefore the damage is repaired without formation of a scar (Silver 1994, Calvin 1998).

Lying between the epidermis and dermis is a thin acellular layer of protein fibres called the 'basement membrane'. Cells of the stratum basale are adherent to one side of this membrane while the other side is attached to the extracellular matrix of the dermis, thus tightly bonding the epidermis and dermis together (Stocum 1995).

The dermis

The dermis is predominantly a connective tissue layer composed of protein fibres called collagen and elastin. The combination of these two fibres gives the dermis a high tensile strength but also flexibility (Bennett & Moody 1995, Tortora & Grabowski 1996). Surrounding these fibres is a complex matrix of dermal proteoglycans that forms a gel-like material called ground substance (Stocum

1995). There are relatively few cells that are normally present in the dermis, however the principal cells are:

- *Fibroblasts* – these cells produce collagen, elastic fibres and ground substance.
- *Macrophages* – these are phagocytic cells important for fighting infection (in their inactivated form they are present in the blood as monocytes and originate in the bone marrow).
- *Mast cells* – these cells are a part of the immune system and release histamine, they are responsible for allergic and hypersensitivity reactions.
- *Adipocytes* – fat cells (Ross *et al.* 1995).

Originating in the dermal layer are the majority of the skin appendages (Fig. 1.1). These accessory structures include:

- *Hair follicles, roots and hair* – hair is found on all parts of the body except for the sides and palms of the hands, sides and soles of the feet, lips and urogenital orifices. The main functions of body hair are protection and thermal regulation;
- *Sebaceous glands* – these are situated at the base of hair follicles and secrete an oily fluid called sebum that travels up hair follicles to the skin. Sebum acts as a waterproofing agent on the skin.
- *Sweat glands* – there are two types of sweat glands. Eccrine glands, present all over the body except the lips, and apocrine glands present only in the axilla, areola, nipple and external genitalia. These glands are a part of the excretion and temperature control systems of the body.
- *Erector pili muscles* – these are tiny muscles attached to the hair follicle and dermis. When they contract they raise hair into a more upright position ('goose-pimples') (Ross *et al.* 1995, Tortora & Grabowski 1996).

As well as these structures, the blood and lymph vessels, and sensory nerve endings of the skin can be found in the dermis. Finger-like projections called dermal papillae extend into the epidermis and contain blood vessels and nerve endings. Hence, the dermis acts as a supporting structure to the epidermis, being responsible for the supply of oxygen and nutrients to this avascular layer (Thomas Hess 1998).

Damage that extends down into the dermis will result in scar formation. The dermis is unable to regenerate itself and any damaged areas are replaced with avascular connective tissue resulting in a scar that is devoid of any skin appendages (Flanagan 1996, Calvin 1998).

The subcutaneous layer

The subcutaneous layer (or hypodermis) is a loose connective tissue composed of adipose and areolar connective tissues. It plays an important role in temperature regulation and energy storage (Ross *et al.* 1995). The depth of this layer is dependent on body site, gender and body composition (Bennett & Moody 1995). This layer contains pressure sensitive nerve endings but only has a minimal blood supply (Tortora & Grabowski 1996). Fibres from the dermis extend into the subcutaneous layer, firmly fixing the skin to it. Because of its poor blood supply, subcutaneous tissue is slow to heal if injured.

Functions of the skin

Skin performs a variety of functions and any damage to, or loss of, skin will affect its ability to carry out these functions effectively. The three main functions of the skin are protection, temperature control and sensation (Mortimer 1998).

Protection

The skin acts as a barrier between the outside environment and the body's internal structures. It does this by preventing the entry of external hazards, such as bacteria and chemicals, and keeping in those substances needed by the body, for example water and electrolytes (Mortimer 1998). The elasticity and toughness of the skin also protects against mechanical injury. Any damage that breaks this barrier acts as a portal for the entry of external material and the loss of internal substances.

Temperature control

Regulation of body temperature is achieved through the skin's extensive blood supply and large surface area in combination with the production of sweat. In a hot environment the blood vessels of the skin dilate to increase the flow of blood and hence heat loss. The evaporation of sweat from the skin's surface enhances this process. In a cold environment blood vessels constrict and reduce the circulation to the skin in order to prevent heat loss. Body hair may stand up (by contraction of the erector pili muscles) to keep a layer of warm air next to the skin (Martin 1996).

1996, Calvin 1998, Moore & Foster 1998b, Thomas Hess 1998, Ehrlich 1999). Some authors also recognise a fourth phase that takes place at the time of injury; this phase is often referred to as haemostasis (Flanagan 2000). Although these phases follow a specific sequence, they do not occur as separate, distinct stages but merge together. The length of each phase depends on the type and nature of the wound.

Haemostasis

As soon as tissue is injured, any damaged blood vessels will constrict to stem the blood flow. In a further attempt to prevent blood loss, the 'coagulation cascade' is initiated by the release of chemical messengers from platelets that have come in contact with collagen from damaged blood vessel walls (Fig. 1.4a) (Olde Damink & Soeters 1997, Silver 1994, Flanagan 2000). Thrombokinase and thromboplastin stimulate the formation of fibrin, while serotonin and adenosine triphosphate promote platelet aggregation (Johnson 1988a). This results in the formation of a fibrin and platelet 'plug' that traps blood cells to form a blood clot and hold the wound edges together (Fig. 1.4b). As this clot loses moisture it dries to form a scab. A blood clot usually forms within five to 10 minutes of an injury occurring (Johnson 1988a, Moore & Foster 1998b).

Inflammation

This phase is sometimes referred to as the destructive phase and is initiated as soon as injury takes place. The release of enzymes from damaged cells results in the breakdown of noradrenaline, which in turn causes dilation of local capillaries and therefore an increased blood flow to the surrounding tissues (Flanagan 1996, Johnson 1988a). Histamine is released from mast cells and increases the permeability of capillaries allowing leakage of fluid into adjacent tissues. Discomfort may occur due to increased pressure on local nerve endings from fluid accumulation. These processes produce the characteristic signs and symptoms of inflammation such as redness, heat, oedema, discomfort and reduced function (Fig. 1.5a) (Flanagan 1999).

Following these initial reactions, the cells involved in healing are attracted to, and start to infiltrate, the damaged area (Fig. 1.5b). Neutrophils arrive in large numbers, their purpose being to attack and destroy any invading bacteria by phagocytosis (ingestion of the foreign body into the cell) to prevent infection (Calvin 1998). As the level of bacterial contamination drops, the predominant

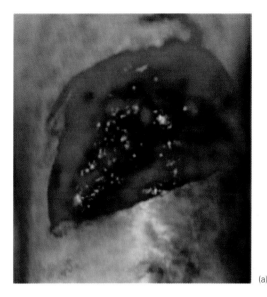

(a)

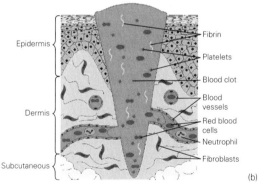

Fig. 1.4
(a) Haemostasis in a
traumatic leg wound; note
blood clots in centre of
wound (photograph kindly
supplied by Dr T.
Fishman.) (b)
Diagrammatic
representation of
haemostasis in a wound
(© Wayne Naylor 2000).

Epidermis

Dermis

Subcutaneous

Fibrin

Platelets

Blood clot

Blood
vessels

Red blood
cells

Neutrophil

Fibroblasts

(b)

cell becomes the macrophage. These cells also remove debris from the wound
through the process of phagocytosis, but their purpose in wound healing is
much more complex than this. The macrophage could be referred to as the 'con-
ductor' of wound healing as it is present for the rest of the healing process and
orchestrates the healing phases (Silver 1994). It does this through the use of

9

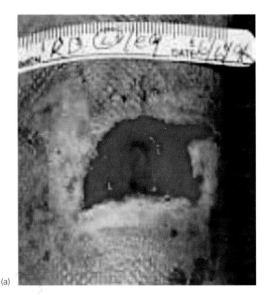

(a)

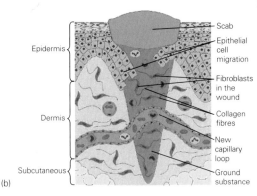

(b)

Epidermis

Dermis

Subcutaneous

Scab

Epithelial cell migration

Fibroblasts in the wound

Collagen fibres

New capillary loop

Ground substance

Fig. 1.6
(a) Formation of granulation tissue during the proliferative phase of healing in a traumatic leg wound (31 days post injury); note the decrease in size of the wound from Fig 1.4a due to wound contraction (Photograph kindly supplied by Dr T. Fishman). (b) Diagrammatic representation of the proliferative phase of wound healing (© Wayne Naylor 2000).

tissue that, in some cases, will be only one-tenth of the size of the original wound (Thomas 1990, Flanagan 1999). Contraction takes place at a rate of 0.6–0.7 mm per day and is not related to wound size; however rectangular wounds do contract more rapidly than round ones (Thomas 1990).

Once the wound has filled with granulation tissue, the process of re-epithelialisation occurs (Fig. 1.6b). Epithelial cells (keratinocytes) usually begin the process of re-epithelialisation within 24 hours of injury (Garrett 1997, Calvin 1998). The epithelial cells may migrate from the wound margin or from hair follicles and sweat glands within the wound itself. How epithelial cells spread across the wound surface is not fully understood and may be by either single cell migration or 'leap-frogging'. Leap-frogging is where a cell moves forward and stops after about four cell lengths, then other cells move over the top of it (Calvin 1998). Individual cells move by extending a pseudopod forward, which attaches to a new position, and then following with the remainder of the cell (amoeboid locomotion). The epithelial cells continue migrating until they come in contact with other epithelial cells (contact inhibition) (Garrett 1997). A moist wound environment has been shown to increase the rate of re-epithelialisation (Eaglstein 1985, Flanagan 1999). New epithelial tissue is pink or white in colour and may appear as small islands within the wound bed.

The proliferative phase may last for up to 24 days, but this will depend on the size of the wound and any factors that may influence healing. Once the wound has filled with new tissue and is covered by epithelium the activity of the macrophages is switched off and the wound moves into the last phase of healing, the maturation, or remodelling, phase.

Maturation

This phase begins at around 21 days after injury and may last from a few months to more than a year (Fig. 1.7a). Events during this phase include a reduction in the number of blood vessels within the new tissue and a reorganisation of collagen bundles along the direction of greatest stress (Silver 1994) (Fig. 1.7b). Remodelling of the collagen bundles also occurs and results in further contraction of the wound; this secondary contraction may result in the formation of contraction deformities, such as those seen after major burns (Silver 1994, Moore & Foster 1998b). The overall purpose of the maturation phase is the replacement of delicate granulation tissue by stronger avascular scar tissue, although this will still only have approximately 70–80% of the strength of normal skin (Calvin 1998, Ehrlich 1999).

Moist wound healing

The original theory of moist wound healing was postulated by Winter (1962) when he found that superficial wounds in pig skin healed faster when kept moist

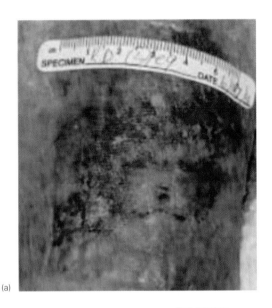

(a)

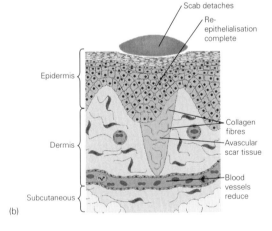

(b)

Scab detaches

Re-epithelialisation complete

Epidermis

Collagen fibres

Dermis

Avascular scar tissue

Blood vessels reduce

Subcutaneous

Fig. 1.7

(a) Maturation phase in a traumatic leg wound (52 days post injury); the wound is now completely covered by new epithelium (Photograph kindly supplied by Dr T. Fishman). (b) Diagrammatic representation of the maturation phase of wound healing (© Wayne Naylor 2000).

under an occlusive dressing than if they were left exposed. He believed that this was due to epithelial cells being able to move freely across the moist wound surface rather than having to burrow underneath a hard scab. Further studies have supported this theory and shown that the synthesis of collagen and formation of new capillaries are also increased in a moist environment (Eaglstein 1985, Dyson *et al.* 1992, Miller 1998a). A moist wound environment may affect the wound in the following ways:

- Increases rate of re-epithelialisation
- Encourages synthesis of collagen and ground substance
- Promotes formation of capillary loops
- Decreases length of inflammatory phase
- Reduces pain and trauma due to dressing adherence
- Promotes breakdown of necrotic tissue (Eaglstein 1985, Dyson *et al.* 1988, Pickworth & De Sousa 1988, Flanagan 1998).

It is generally accepted that a moist wound environment is ideal for wound healing (Table 1.1). The moist environment is usually achieved through the use of occlusive dressings such as hydrocolloids and semi-permeable films. A common misconception is that these dressings may promote wound infection; however, evidence has shown that occlusive dressings do not increase the rate of wound infection (Hutchinson & Lawrence 1991, Williams & Young 1998).

FACTORS THAT INFLUENCE WOUND HEALING

There are a number of factors that may influence the healing process. These may be either external or internal in nature and will affect wound healing in a

Table 1.1 The ideal wound healing environment.

The ideal wound healing environment should:
- Be moist but free of excess exudate
- Be free from slough, necrotic tissue and foreign bodies
- Prevent further trauma, for example by adherence of dressing products or from external sources such as pressure or friction
- Keep the wound at body temperature (37°C)
- Protect the wound from external contamination by pathogens, toxic substances or debris
- Be acidic (a slightly acidic environment accelerates healing)
- Allow gaseous exchange

Table 1.2 Factors that influence wound healing.

Factor	Effect on wound healing	Prevention/amelioration
Mechanical stress	Includes pressure, friction and shear. Pressure will reduce capillary blood flow resulting in a lack of oxygen and nutrients reaching the wound. Friction is produced as the skin slides over another surface. This may result in damage to, or even removal of, new tissue. Shear is caused when the skin is forced in the opposite direction to underlying structures to which it is attached. The forces produced can damage newly formed tissue that lacks tensile strength (Cutting 1994)	Appropriate lifting and repositioning of patient and use of pressure relieving equipment. Use of low friction and shear surfaces (Laverty *et al.* 2000a). Irrigate wound rather than swab with low-linting gauze
Wound site	Wounds in areas of high vascularity, such as the head and neck, often heal better than those in less vascular sites, such as the pre-tibial area. A wound over a joint or other highly mobile area may also take longer to heal due to the constant movement (Benbow 1995)	Immobilise joints if necessary and/or use flexible dressing products
Wound temperature	If the temperature of the wound drops below body temperature then cellular activity decreases, thereby slowing healing. Frequent dressing changes, use of irrigation fluid at room temperature or leaving the wound exposed will all result in a drop in wound temperature (Collier 1996)	Maintain wound at body temperature. Leave dressing in place for as long as possible; use thermally insulating dressings (foams, hydrocolloids). Use warm (preferably body temperature) 0.9% sodium chloride for irrigation and do not leave the wound exposed for long periods (e.g. for ward rounds)

Table 1.2 *Continued*

Factor	Effect on wound healing	Prevention/amelioration
Desiccation	Wounds that are allowed to dry out have a longer inflammatory phase and are slower to heal than wounds maintained in a moist environment (Dyson *et al.* 1988)	Maintain a moist wound environment
Maceration	Excess moisture in and around the wound (exudate, urine or sweat) may cause breakdown of adjacent skin and enlargement of the wound	Use a dressing product that will absorb excess exudate and use a skin barrier to protect surrounding healthy skin
Infection	The release of proteases by infecting organisms re-injures tissues within the wound and may prolong the inflammatory phase (Bowler 1998, Thomson 1998). Bacteria may also compete with macrophages and fibroblasts for available oxygen and nutrients (Cutting 1994)	Hand washing and use of aseptic or clean technique when treating wounds. Use occlusive dressings to protect wound from external pathogens
Medications	Steroid and rheumatoid drugs reduce the inflammatory response. Steroid use over a long time may also suppress fibroblasts and, therefore, collagen synthesis and wound strength (Bale & Jones 1997, Moore & Foster 1998b). Wound contraction and epithelialisation may also be affected (Bland *et al.* 1984) Chemotherapy (cytotoxic drugs) can adversely affect wound healing by inhibiting cell division and protein synthesis (Bland *et al.* 1984). It may also induce immunosuppression, hence delaying the inflammatory response (Lotti *et al.* 1998) Immunosuppressants reduce white blood cell activity (neutrophils and macrophages), delaying the inflammatory phase and autolytic wound cleansing. They may also increase the risk of wound infection	Systemic or local vitamin A may counteract the anti-inflammatory effects of steroids. Review use of steroid therapies

Aseptic technique for wound care, use of protective occlusive dressings |

Table 1.2 *Continued*

Factor	Effect on wound healing	Prevention/amelioration
	Antibiotics prevent or treat wound infections, thereby enhancing wound healing (Cutting 1994)	
Radiotherapy	Affects cell reproduction, thereby delaying healing. May cause damage to local capillaries and basal cells resulting in a localised skin reaction and possibly the formation of a superficial wound (Sitton 1992). Wound healing is usually delayed in areas that have been irradiated due to capillary damage (Sussman 1998)	Some form of skin reaction is usually unavoidable but the use of moisturisers or emollient creams may delay skin breakdown. Avoid irradiating an existing wound if possible (however radiotherapy may be indicated for malignant wounds)
Malignancy	Along with primary skin lesions and anticancer therapies, there are a number of adverse effects related to malignant tumours. These include malnutrition, altered coagulation (disseminated intravascular coagulation), and altered angiogenesis and re-epithelialisation (Lotti *et al.* 1998)	Malnutrition may be managed as outlined below (nutritional state). However, the other effects of malignancies are difficult, if not impossible, to prevent
Wound care	Topical antiseptics can delay healing by damaging normal cells (Gilchrist 1999)	Use 0.9% sodium chloride or water for wound irrigation
	Inappropriate use of dressing products may also impede healing by adhering to the wound bed or keeping the wound too wet or too dry. Frequent dressing changes or use of products outside of the manufacturers' recommendations may also have adverse effects on healing	Careful assessment of the wound and selection of a dressing that matches the needs of the wound and the patient
Lifestyle	The two main factors are smoking and alcohol abuse. Smoking reduces the ability of haemoglobin to carry oxygen and also causes peripheral vasoconstriction resulting in a lack of	Encourage patient to reduce or stop smoking and alcohol use, and promote a balanced nutritional diet. This may

Table 1.2 *Continued*

Factor	Effect on wound healing	Prevention/amelioration
	oxygen and nutrients to the wound (Moore & Foster 1998b). It may also increase the risk of clot formation by increasing platelet aggregation (Bale & Jones 1997, Williams & Young 1998) Excessive alcohol use can damage the liver leading to clotting problems. Malnutrition is also common in alcoholics (Cutting 1994)	need referral for specialist help and support, for example to a dietician
General health	Underlying health problems can affect the blood supply to the wound and the inflammatory response. For example peripheral vascular disease, heart disease, diabetes and arteriosclerosis will impede the blood supply. Diabetes and immune disorders may delay or reduce the normal inflammatory response to injury	Accurate assessment and treatment of underlying health problems will reduce their impact on wound healing
Age	There is a reduction in the elasticity of elderly skin making it more fragile. The healing process is also slowed down due to a reduced metabolic rate and poor circulation (Bale & Jones 1997) Problems with nutrition, impaired mobility and mental or physical illnesses may also impact on wound healing in older people (Mahony 1999)	Ageing of the skin is unavoidable but careful skin and wound care can reduce the risk of skin damage and infection.
Nutritional state	Adequate nutrition is vital for wound healing. Malnutrition can result in delayed healing due to a lack of essential nutrients including protein, carbohydrates, fats, vitamins and trace elements. Dehydration will also adversely affect healing by disturbing cellular metabolism and reducing circulatory blood volume. Malnourished patients are also at an increased risk of	Identification and assessment of individuals at risk of malnutrition and development of an appropriate nutritional support plan. It is essential to involve a dietician in the patient's care. The use of enteral (percutaneous

Table 1.2 *Continued*

Factor	Effect on wound healing	Prevention/amelioration
	infection because of a reduced immune response (Wells 1994, Olde Damink & Soeters 1997)	endoscopic gastrostomy or nasogastric tube) or parenteral (intravenous total parenteral nutrition) feeding may be necessary
Body composition	Obesity can influence healing by reducing the availability of oxygen to the skin, increasing the risk of post-operative infection and haematoma formation and excoriation of the skin in skin folds (Armstrong 1998) Patients who are underweight also experience problems due to protein being used for metabolism rather than in the production of new tissue (Cutting 1994)	Dietary assessment and advice as above. Appropriate skin and pressure area care.
Psychological	Some studies have reported that stress may inhibit the growth of fibroblasts (Moore & Foster 1998b). Stress can also adversely affect the immune system causing a delay in healing (Kiecolt-Glaser *et al.* 1995). Inadequate sleep may also affect wound healing (Adam & Oswald 1983, Bale & Jones 1997).	The psychological state of the patient should be included as part of a holistic wound assessment. To help reduce anxiety, ensure the patient is fully informed about any treatments that they are receiving and that they have an opportunity to discuss any concerns. A referral for psychological support may be appropriate.

variety of ways. Some of the more notable factors are nutrition, infection, age, mechanical stress and drug therapies (Moore & Foster 1998b, Cutting 1994, Miller & Dyson 1996, Bale & Jones 1997). These factors along with several others are listed in Table 1.2, together with their effect on the healing wound.

CONCLUSION

Maintaining or restoring the integrity of the skin is important not only for aesthetic reasons but also to maintain its essential homeostatic and protective functions. The combined knowledge of wound healing physiology and the factors that may affect healing will make it possible to develop an effective wound management strategy in order to restore tissue integrity. An important part of this management plan is accurate wound assessment, which will elicit the stage of healing and highlight any deviations from the norm that may be caused by underlying factors. Wounds that do not follow the normal healing phases may take considerable time to heal, or, as is the case with wounds caused by a malignancy, may not heal at all. These chronic wounds can be complex in their management and stretch the abilities of even very experienced health care professionals.

2 Wound Assessment

PRINCIPLES OF ASSESSMENT

Introduction

The nursing process provides a dynamic and logical method in which the nurse may sensitively and systematically approach nursing practice to achieve mutually determined goals with the patient, thus ensuring that the care given is appropriate and effective (Fig. 2.1). This process is reliant upon critical thinking, decision-making, clinical judgement, observation and interpersonal skills (Pennery *et al.* 2000).

Nursing assessment

Accurate assessment is vital in order to provide correct treatment and care, and to evaluate the effectiveness of interventions and treatments. The initial identification and assessment of the patient's actual and/or potential needs, problems and expectations, provide baseline information against which new and changing information can be compared. The use of a conceptual nursing model that integrates concepts and statements into a meaningful framework, for example Roper, Logan and Tierney's Activities of Daily Living, will be helpful as a means of holistic patient assessment (Collier 1994, Moore 1997a).

General patient assessment should, in most cases, come first and, at a minimum, include the information presented in Table 2.1. This data may be collected from a number of sources including the patient's notes, the patient themselves or the patient's family or carer. For patients in hospital or a hospice much of this information may already have been collected during the initial nursing and medical admission assessments.

Assessment that elicits the deeper meaning of superficial cues and includes the meanings attributed to events by the patient, is associated with greater diagnostic accuracy and thus more effective intervention (Gordon 1994). Also, focusing upon the patient's perception of function in their activities of daily life, together with other significant persons, is crucial in the identification of needs (Ehrenberg *et al.* 1996). This aspect of assessment was highlighted in a recent

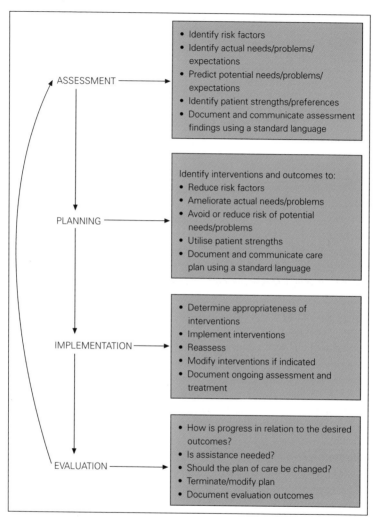

Fig. 2.1 Dynamic nursing process as used by a critical thinker (adapted from Alfaro-Lefevre 1999).

Table 2.1 Parameters of general patient assessment.

(1) Past health history, disease status, previous/current medical treatment
(2) Nutritional status, such as obesity or malnutrition
(3) Any information needs or concerns of the patient or their family/carers (i.e. understanding of their illness)
(4) Patient strengths and coping abilities
(5) Previous experiences of illness and the meaning of these experiences to the patient
(6) Sleep and rest
(7) Mobility which may affect circulation and predispose to pressure ulcers
(8) Psychological issues should be addressed and subjects such as depression, body image, stress and sexuality may be included
(9) Social support/resources need to be ascertained for discharge planning
(10) Spiritual and cultural needs

study where differences were noted between nurses' and patients' views of the patients' needs while in hospital (Lauri *et al.* 1997). Another important point is that assessment should include the patient's own concerns, feelings and preferences (Moore 1997a). This is essential in order to provide an individualised and patient-centred care plan, especially for patients with complex and/or chronic non-healing wounds.

Identifying the impact of any symptoms upon the patient's life, such as distress, social isolation, relationship problems, and the ability of the patient to function 'normally' (e.g. ability to go to work, care for children, leisure, self-care ability), is imperative in an holistic assessment. Information regarding past and present social and psychological functioning and the level of medical and social support will assist when developing a plan of care.

Communication

Therapeutic verbal and non-verbal communication is key to successful patient assessment and can be used to establish rapport (Mallett 1997, Pennery *et al.* 2000). This may facilitate the expression of the patient's needs and recognises the importance of regarding patients as individuals with unique expectations and problems. Multidisciplinary communication is also paramount and in the UK the use of the term 'patient needs/problems' encompasses the concept that care may involve collaboration from disciplines other than nursing. The use of a standard language to describe patient needs, problems and interventions for which nurses and other health professionals assume accountability will facilitate communication, documentation and continuity of care (Leih & Salentijn 1994).

ASSESSING THE PATIENT WITH A WOUND

For chronic and/or complex wounds examination of the local wound environment is the third priority in assessment, and should take place following assessment of the patient's general health status and underlying causes of the wound (Casey 1997, Flanagan 1997, Miller 1999).

General patient assessment has been extensively covered elsewhere and in particular may be achieved through the use of the many published nursing assessment frameworks. Therefore the main focus of this chapter will be on assessment of the local wound environment.

Wound assessment charts

The use of documentation to assist in the assessment process is recommended to facilitate continuity of care and appropriate evaluation of all relevant areas and to fulfil legal and professional requirements (Collier 1994, Benbow 1995, Sterling 1996, Flanagan 1997, Moore 1997a, Miller 1999, Bachand & McNicholas 1999). There are numerous assessment charts available and some centres use a combination of several. The aim of the documentation is to provide an accessible reference for members of the multidisciplinary team, including patients or carers, detailing the present and previous assessment and management of the wound.

In a study that compared the use of a wound assessment chart to no chart, it was found that when a chart was available nurses were more likely to document wound assessments and less likely to use irrelevant and biased statements (Sterling 1996). An example of an assessment form that has been used for fungating wounds, and which addressed both the physical and psychological aspects, is the TELER system. This assessment tool utilises an ordinal scale scoring system to measure outcomes of patient care and was used to evaluate the effectiveness of wound care products in controlling the symptoms of fungating wounds (Grocott 1998).

When selecting a wound assessment tool the following points should be taken into consideration (see also p. 30):
- Is it easy to use (i.e. not complicated or too long)?
- Does it meet the needs of the specific patient group?
- Do all team members understand it?

RMH WOUND ASSESSMENT CHART

INITIAL ASSESSMENT

Fill in all spaces that apply to the patient with either a tick or text

THE ROYAL
MARSDEN

Patient details: Date of initial assessment: _____	**Factors that may delay healing:**
Patient name: _____	Infection _____
Hospital number: _____ Age: _____	Diabetes _____
	Anaemia/neutropenia HGB= WBC=
Diagnosis: _____	Immobility _____
Current Treatment: _____	Over/under weight _____
_____	Poor nutritional status _____
Medications (specify): _____	Poor sleep and rest _____
	Alcohol/tobacco use _____
Allergies: _____	Previous radiotherapy _____
Length of time wound present: ___ days/weeks/months*	Underlying disease _____
(*delete as appropriate)	(e.g. vascular disease)

Wound is due to:	**Wound dimensions:**	**Wound bed (approximate % cover):**
Tumour involvement ☐	Max length (cm) _____	Necrotic (BLACK) _____
Radiotherapy induced ☐		
Pressure ☐	Max width (cm) _____	Slough (YELLOW) _____
Surgical complications ☐		
Vascular disease ☐	Max depth (cm) _____	Granulating (RED) _____
Trauma ☐		
Other (please state) ☐	Surface area (cm²)	Epithelialising (PINK) _____

Exudate level:	**Bleeding:**	**Pain from wound (see part (d)):**
None ☐	None ☐	Level (0–10 using VAS) _____
Low ☐	Slight ☐	Continuous _____
Moderate ☐	Moderate ☐	At specific times (list) _____
High ☐	Heavy ☐	
Type of exudate (e.g.	At dressing change ☐	Current analgesia _____
serous, bloodstained, pus)		

Skin around wound:	**Odour (see part (d)):**	*Type of Pain*	
		Stinging	☐
	None ☐	Stabbing	☐
Intact ☐	Slight ☐	Aching	☐
Healthy ☐	Moderate ☐	Throbbing	☐
Fragile ☐	Strong ☐	Itching	☐
Dry ☐		Other (specify)	☐
Scaly ☐			
Erythema ☐	**Location (mark diagram):**	**Referrals (name and date):**
Maceration ☐		Clinical nurse
Oedema ☐		specialist _____
Eczema ☐		
Skin nodules ☐		Pharmacist _____
Skin stripping ☐	Right ... Left Left ... Right	Dietician _____
Dressing allergy ☐		
Tape allergy ☐		Surgeon _____
Other (please state) ☐		Other (state) _____

Assessed by (sign and print name):

(a)

Fig. 2.2 Wound assessment chart.

Diagram of wound if appropriate (or attach tracing/photograph):

Indicate dimensions and orientation of wound and the type and size of tissue present

Date: _____	Date: _____
Date: _____	Date: _____
Date: _____	Date: _____

(b)

Fig. 2.2 *Continued*

Ongoing assessment						
Date of Assessment (weekly)						
Wound dimensions						
Max length (cm)						
Max width (cm)						
Max depth (cm)						
Surface area (cm²)						
Wound bed – approximate % cover (enter %)						
Necrotic (BLACK)						
Slough (YELLOW)						
Granulating (RED)						
Epithelialising (PINK)						
Skin around wound						
Intact						
Healthy						
Fragile						
Dry						
Scaly						
Erythema						
Maceration						
Oedema						
Eczema						
Skin nodules						
Skin stripping						
Dressing allergy						
Tape allergy						
Other (please state)						
Exudate level						
None						
Low						
Moderate						
High						
Amount increasing						
Amount decreasing						
Odour (see scale in (d))						
None						
Slight						
Moderate						
Strong						
Bleeding						
None						
Slight						
Moderate						
Heavy						
At dressing change						
Pain from wound (using Visual Analogue Scale – part (d))						
Level (0–10)						
Continuous						
At specific times (specify)						
Interventions for pain (analgesia/ pain relief)						
Wound infection suspected						
Swab taken (Y/N)						
Swab result						
Treatment						
Assessment review date						
Initials of Assessor						

(c)

Fig. 2.2 *Continued*

Wound management plan		
Date /Time	**Wound management plan (cleansing/dressings) ⇨ Complete if plan altered**	**Signature (print name)**

Visual Analogue Scale (VAS) for patient's rating of pain

Place a mark at on the line at the point that best describes your pain

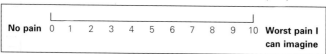

No pain 0 1 2 3 4 5 6 7 8 9 10 **Worst pain I can imagine**

Rating Scale for Odour (adapted from Baker & Haig 1981 and Poteete 1993)

Score	Assessment
None	No odour evident, even when at the patient's bedside with the dressing removed
Slight	Wound odour is evident at close proximity to the patient when the dressing is removed
Moderate	Wound odour is evident upon entering the room (1.5–3 m from patient) with the dressing removed
Strong	Wound odour is evident upon entering the room (1.5–3 m from patient) with the dressing intact

(d)

Fig. 2.2 *Continued*

- Has its reliability and validity been tested?
- Is it based on research or other reliable evidence (such as expert opinion)?
- Does it assist in the identification of treatment or care objectives?
- Does it help to identify wound improvements/deterioration?

(Flanagan 1997, Moore 1997a)

Figure 2.2 is a wound assessment chart that has been designed for use in an oncology setting. This chart has been developed from expert nursing opinion, internal hospital audit results and a literature review of wound assessment and wound healing in oncology patients (including fungating wounds and radio-therapy skin reactions). The reliability and validity of this chart is currently being evaluated.

Parameters of assessment

There are a variety of parameters that should be included when assessing the local wound environment in order to plan the most appropriate management. However, care needs to be taken when evaluating some of these parameters, as measurements may be open to individual interpretation, for example exudate, odour and bleeding. The major difficulty in assessing these symptoms is a lack of valid and reliable measures. When a scale or scoring system is used it is important that the professionals using it agree on whether the indicators are recorded as relative to the previous state of the wound or relative to another wound of similar shape, size and aetiology. Comparison of the assessment data to previous data on the same wound will reduce the possibility of measurements being based on the assessor's past experiences and show trends and changes in the state of the wound. However, comparison to another similar wound may assist in appropriate dressing product selection. Some aspects of the wound can only be assessed via observation, such as the type of tissue present, colour of exudate and size of the wound. Once again it is important to have a standardised and valid method of measuring and recording these parameters to ensure inter-rater reliability.

Local wound assessment

Following the general assessment the focus turns to the local wound environment. There are a number of aspects that should be considered but the importance of each will vary between wounds. This assessment should provide the practitioner with the necessary information on which to base the selection of wound management products or the need for other local or systemic treatments. Parameters to include in the local wound assessment are listed below.

(1) Aetiology or cause of wound

It is important to know the cause of the wound so that treatment can be planned accordingly. For example if it is a fungating wound, care is directed towards symptom control, or if the wound is related to radiotherapy it will not heal until treatment has been completed.

(2) Location

The location of the wound may affect the rate of healing and will also influence the choice of dressing. It may also indicate the cause of the wound, e.g. pressure ulcer or a wound within a radiotherapy field, and potential complications, such as haemorrhage.

(3) Size, depth and shape

The emphasis on measuring the wound is to monitor changes in size. This is principally to provide evidence of wound healing or deterioration and the effectiveness of wound management strategies. Measurements should include the surface area and volume of the wound if possible (Collier 1994, Flanagan 1997, Moore 1997b, Miller 1999). There are a number of methods suggested for measuring wound size including acetate tracings, rulers, photography, alginate cavity fillers, computer mapping, structured light, laser triangulation and ultrasound (Collier 1994). The last five are not generally used in everyday clinical practice except perhaps computer mapping using digital photography which is becoming popular and more accessible to many practitioners. However, for everyday use it is currently more usual to employ a combination of manual measurements, such as tracing or ruler, and photography (Vowden 1995).

(4) Amount and nature of exudate

A certain amount of exudate is normal during the healing process and it is important that the wound is kept in a moist environment. Excess exudate can indicate infection, especially if it has a yellow, green or grey colour, and can lead to maceration and breakdown of the skin surrounding the wound (Moore 1997b, Flanagan 1994). The amount and type of exudate present should be recorded.

Generally indicators such as 'low', 'medium' and 'high' are used to assess the amount of exudate. However, exudate should be measured and documented relative to the previous state of the wound and any increase or decrease in amount should be taken into account in order to assess the success or otherwise of interventions (see Fig. 2.2c). Nevertheless, a measurement should also be made relative to other, similar wounds in order to ensure the most appropriate dressing is chosen. Some additional methods of measuring exudate include weighing dressings, recording the number of dressing changes over a specific time period or using a drainable wound manager or ostomy appliance to collect exudate. The latter could be the most accurate. Unfortunately the difficulty in recording wound drainage will continue until a reliable, valid and simple method of measuring exudate production is described.

(5) Odour

Statements such as 'none', 'mild' and 'offensive' are commonly used to rate odour but these measures may be influenced by previous experiences of the assessor and it may be more appropriate to use a descriptive rating scale (Fig. 2.3). Any increase or decrease in odour should also be noted as this is related to wound infection or changes in the type of wound discharge (e.g. faecal). Generally though, the presence of malodour is difficult to assess impartially and therefore self-assessment by the patient may be more appropriate (Collier 1997) (see Fig. 2.4).

(6) Type of tissue present

The type of tissue present in the wound will impact on the choice of dressing and depends on how the tissue present should be managed. For example,

None	– No odour evident, even when at the patient's bedside with the dressing removed
Slight	– Wound odour is evident at close proximity to the patient when the dressing is removed
Moderate	– Wound odour is evident upon entering the room (1.5–3 m from patient) with the dressing removed
Strong	– Wound odour is evident upon entering the room (1.5–3 m from patient) with the dressing intact

Fig. 2.3 Odour assessment scale (Baker & Haig 1981, Poteete 1993).

necrotic or sloughy wounds need a dressing that will debride the dead tissue. A number of authors suggest using various 'colour coding' for the determination of tissue type at the wound base. Flanagan (1997) suggests a four-colour classification system: black (necrotic), yellow (sloughy), red (granulating) and pink (epithelialising). A five-colour system has also been proposed and includes green for infected wounds (Collier 1994, Benbow 1995).

(7) Signs of infection
The presence of infection is usually observed via local and systemic signs and symptoms including swelling, heat and redness at the wound site, and

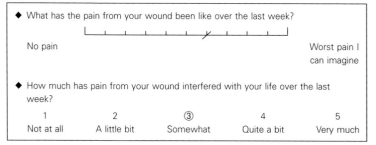

Wound Symptoms Self-Assessment Chart (WoSSAC)

Instructions to Patient
This short questionnaire will help us to manage any problems you may be having because of your wound. Twenty-one problems have been listed and we would like you to indicate the scale of each problem for you as well as how much it is interfering with your life.

There are two parts to each question. For the first part place a mark on the line at the point that best describes the problem for you. For the second part circle a number to show how much you feel a problem has interfered with your life over the last week.

Answer each question as best you can. There are no right or wrong answers.

Here is an example

◆ What has the pain from your wound been like over the last week?

No pain   Worst pain I
                                                     can imagine

◆ How much has pain from your wound interfered with your life over the last week?

1	2	③	4	5
Not at all	A little bit	Somewhat	Quite a bit	Very much

Fig. 2.4 The Wound Symptoms Self-Assessment Chart (WoSSAC) (© Wayne Naylor 2000).

1.

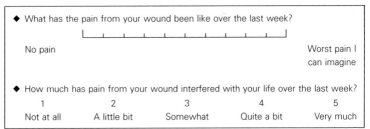

What has the pain from your wound been like over the last week?

No pain   Worst pain I can imagine

How much has pain from your wound interfered with your life over the last week?

1	2	3	4	5
Not at all	A little bit	Somewhat	Quite a bit	Very much

2.

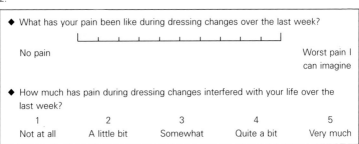

What has your pain been like during dressing changes over the last week?

No pain   Worst pain I can imagine

How much has pain during dressing changes interfered with your life over the last week?

1	2	3	4	5
Not at all	A little bit	Somewhat	Quite a bit	Very much

3.

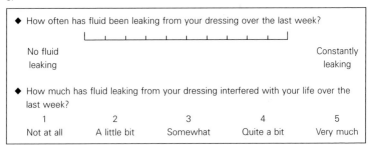

How often has fluid been leaking from your dressing over the last week?

No fluid leaking   Constantly leaking

How much has fluid leaking from your dressing interfered with your life over the last week?

1	2	3	4	5
Not at all	A little bit	Somewhat	Quite a bit	Very much

Fig. 2.4 *Continued*

4.

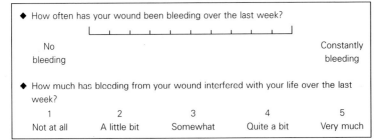

◆ How often has your wound been bleeding over the last week?

No bleeding	Constantly bleeding

◆ How much has bleeding from your wound interfered with your life over the last week?

1	2	3	4	5
Not at all	A little bit	Somewhat	Quite a bit	Very much

5.

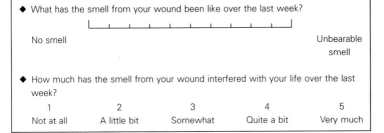

◆ What has the smell from your wound been like over the last week?

No smell	Unbearable smell

◆ How much has the smell from your wound interfered with your life over the last week?

1	2	3	4	5
Not at all	A little bit	Somewhat	Quite a bit	Very much

6.

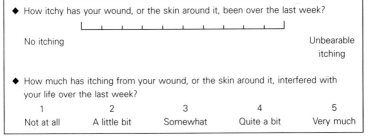

◆ How itchy has your wound, or the skin around it, been over the last week?

No itching	Unbearable itching

◆ How much has itching from your wound, or the skin around it, interfered with your life over the last week?

1	2	3	4	5
Not at all	A little bit	Somewhat	Quite a bit	Very much

Fig. 2.4 *Continued*

7.

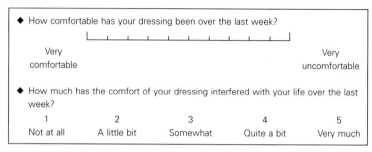

8.

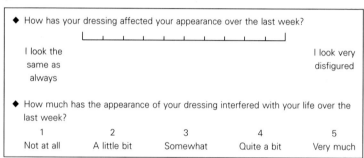

9.

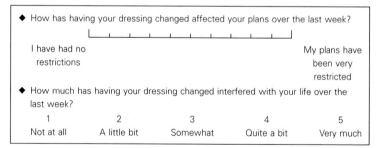

Fig. 2.4 *Continued*

10.

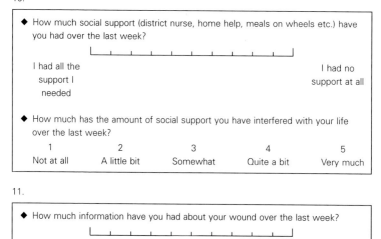

◆ How much social support (district nurse, home help, meals on wheels etc.) have
  you had over the last week?

I had all the				I had no
support I				support at all
needed				

◆ How much has the amount of social support you have interfered with your life
  over the last week?

1	2	3	4	5
Not at all	A little bit	Somewhat	Quite a bit	Very much

11.

◆ How much information have you had about your wound over the last week?

I had all the				I had no
information I				information
needed				at all

◆ How much has needing information about your wound interfered with your life
  over the last week?

1	2	3	4	5
Not at all	A little bit	Somewhat	Quite a bit	Very much

12.

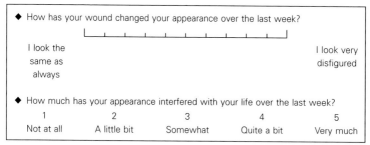

◆ How has your wound changed your appearance over the last week?

I look the				I look very
same as				disfigured
always				

◆ How much has your appearance interfered with your life over the last week?

1	2	3	4	5
Not at all	A little bit	Somewhat	Quite a bit	Very much

Fig. 2.4 *Continued*

13.

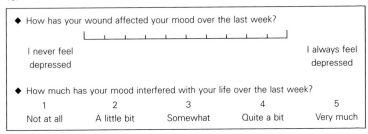

♦ How has your wound affected your mood over the last week?

I never feel
depressed

I always feel
depressed

♦ How much has your mood interfered with your life over the last week?

1	2	3	4	5
Not at all	A little bit	Somewhat	Quite a bit	Very much

14.

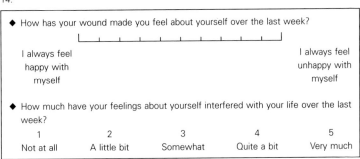

♦ How has your wound made you feel about yourself over the last week?

I always feel
happy with
myself

I always feel
unhappy with
myself

♦ How much have your feelings about yourself interfered with your life over the last week?

1	2	3	4	5
Not at all	A little bit	Somewhat	Quite a bit	Very much

15.

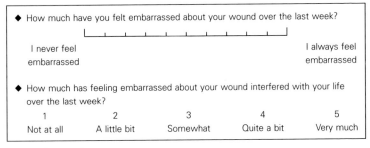

♦ How much have you felt embarrassed about your wound over the last week?

I never feel
embarrassed

I always feel
embarrassed

♦ How much has feeling embarrassed about your wound interfered with your life over the last week?

1	2	3	4	5
Not at all	A little bit	Somewhat	Quite a bit	Very much

Fig. 2.4 *Continued*

16.

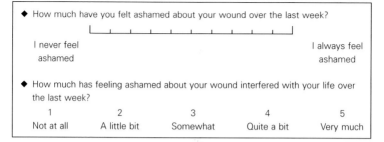

17.

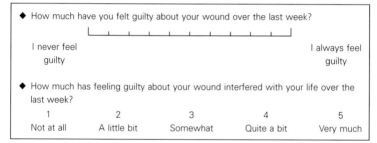

18.

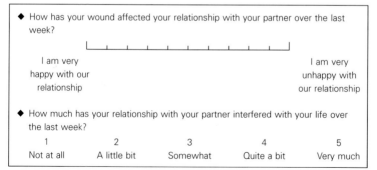

Fig. 2.4 *Continued*

19.

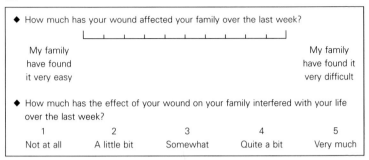

20.

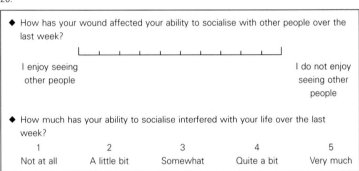

21.

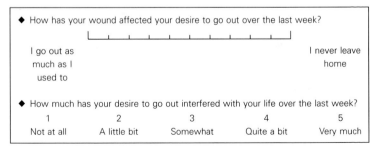

Fig. 2.4 *Continued*

WoSSAC Symptom Evaluation Grid

INSTRUCTIONS FOR USE

Fill in the Grid for each symptom once the patient has completed the self-assessment chart. For severity record the level by counting the number of lines from left (0) to the patient's mark and then colour in an equal number of blocks. Record the level of interference (circled number) in the box below the severity scale (see example).

Patient Name: _____

Hospital Number: _____

Ward: _____
(or affix Patient Label)

Example

	0 1 2 3 4 5 6 7 8 9 10				
1	2	③	4	5
Not at all	A little bit	Somewhat	Quite a bit	Very much

	DATE	0/00											
EXAMPLE	Severity	■											
	Interference	3											

	DATE												
1. PAIN FROM WOUND	Severity												
	Interference												
2. PAIN DURING DRESSING CHANGE	Severity												
	Interference												
3. LEAKAGE OF EXUDATE	Severity												
	Interference												
4. BLEEDING FROM WOUND	Severity												
	Interference												
5. SMELL FROM WOUND	Severity												
	Interference												
6. ITCHING RELATED TO WOUND	Severity												
	Interference												
7. COMFORT OF DRESSING	Severity												
	Interference												

Fig. 2.4 *Continued*

41

8. APPEARANCE OF DRESSING	Severity														
	Interference														
9. RESTRICTIONS ON LIFE	Severity														
	Interference														
10. SOCIAL SUPPORT	Severity														
	Interference														
11. INFORMATION NEEDS	Severity														
	Interference														
12. APPEARANCE	Severity														
	Interference														
13. DEPRESSION (MOOD)	Severity														
	Interference														
14. FEELINGS ABOUT SELF (SELF-ESTEEM)	Severity														
	Interference														
15. FEELING EMBARRASSED	Severity														
	Interference														
16. FEELING ASHAMED	Severity														
	Interference														
17. FEELING GUILTY	Severity														
	Interference														
18. RELATIONSHIP WITH PARTNER	Severity														
	Interference														
19. EFFECT ON FAMILY	Severity														
	Interference														
20. ABILITY TO SOCIALISE	Severity														
	Interference														
21. DESIRE TO GO OUT	Severity														
	Interference														
Assessed by (initials)															

Please file the WoSSAC Symptom Evaluation Grid in the patient's nursing notes

Fig. 2.4 *Continued*

generalised pyrexia (Benbow 1995, Miller 1996). However, increases in patient reported symptoms such as pain, exudate and odour levels may also indicate an infection, particularly in patients who are immunosuppressed or who have chronic wounds (Gilchrist 1999).

(8) Nature and type of pain
Pain is often undervalued by professionals and the rating of a patient's pain may be affected by preconceived assumptions of the assessor (Moore 1997b). Therefore the use of a patient self-assessment, such as a visual analogue scale, is recommended (Collier 1997) (see Figs 2.3 and 2.4). There is also a need for appropriate pain assessment parameters, which may include nature, severity, site, frequency, impact on daily living and effectiveness of treatments (Collier 1994, Benbow 1995, Sterling 1996).

(9) Pain related to dressing changes and wound cleansing
The type of dressing or cleansing technique used can contribute to pain during dressing changes (Hollinworth 1997). Dressings such as gauze or paraffin impregnated tulle may adhere to the wound bed causing tissue damage and pain on removal. Swabbing a wound during cleansing or the use of high-pressure irrigation or certain cleansing products can also cause pain and damage new tissue. Using cold irrigation fluid may also exacerbate pain (Hollinworth 1997). Therefore the presence of pain may be an important indicator that there is a need for change in the dressing regime.

(10) Condition of surrounding skin
The appearance of the skin surrounding the wound can indicate the presence of infection (heat, redness, oedema) or dressing/tape allergies (Benbow 1995, Collier 1994). Fragile, sensitive or macerated skin may need protection with 'skin barriers' and it may be necessary to avoid the use of adhesives.

(11) Episodes of bleeding
Episodes of bleeding may indicate erosion of underlying blood vessels, particularly in fungating wounds, especially if bleeding is spontaneous and heavy. Dressing removal may also cause bleeding if fragile tissue is damaged by adherent dressings.

(12) Other factors
Any other factors that may affect healing of the wound or the choice of dressing product should be recorded. This includes information such as fistula or sinus leakage, proximity of a stoma and current or previous treatments that may affect healing, for example radiotherapy or steroid therapy.

Once the local wound assessment has been performed the information obtained should be documented in the nursing care plan along with the cleansing and dressing regime chosen to manage the wound.

Assessment of complex/chronic wounds

The importance of a full and comprehensive assessment cannot be over-emphasised when one considers the potential effect of chronic or complex wound symptoms on the patient's life. A chronic wound is one that does not heal as expected according to the 'normal' process of wound healing. It is usually of long duration with slow changes and associated with an underlying disease process. A complex wound, which may not necessarily be chronic, is one that is associated with multiple pathology and/or multiple symptoms and requires specialised assessment and management interventions. Fungating wounds, high-grade pressure ulcers, complicated plastic surgery wounds and chronic leg ulcers fit into these categories as they are related to an underlying disease, have multiple associated symptoms and/or require specialised care. In addition, fungating wounds will rarely heal and, because they are relatively uncommon in most health care settings, are often outside of most health care professionals' experience.

The nature of complex and chronic wounds makes each one unique. Symptoms may vary considerably between patients and the significance of each symptom will be interpreted differently by different patients. Therefore the impact of the wound on the patient's quality of life is highly individual. When assessing chronic/complex wounds it is important to identify any existent and/or potential problems. This should be from the patient's or carer's perspective but should also include the health care professional's opinion. Although physical problems are frequently focused on, psychosocial issues and their impact on the patient's life are of equal, if not more, importance. One way of evaluating the impact of a wound on a patient's life is to ask the patient to rate his or her own symptoms. Figure 2.4 is a patient self-assessment tool that was developed specifically for use by patients with fungating wounds.

This tool was developed from an extensive literature review on fungating wounds, wound assessment and symptom self-assessment scales. It asks the patient to rate 21 symptoms and problems related to their wound using visual analogue scales for severity of the symptom or problem and Likert scales for interference with the patient's life (Naylor 2000). These scores are then recorded on a symptom evaluation grid that gives an ongoing visual record and provides a means of monitoring the effectiveness of interventions. Preliminary work suggests that this tool has a high level of validity; however clinical studies are planned with more in-depth analysis to fully evaluate its reliability and validity.

Assessment of the patient will be ongoing and the likelihood is that the symptoms and consequent plan of care will change as circumstances dictate. For example, issues relating to changes in body image may be ongoing and dependent on where the patient is in regard to their acceptance and coping with their diagnosis and/or prognosis. Patients and their carers must be given encouragement to participate in this process and raise issues when they become pertinent to them. Being able to ask the patient's opinions of their symptoms and consequent management is time saving and beneficial. It also demonstrates to the patient that their input is valid and appreciated.

CONCLUSION

Wound assessment is important for many reasons and should not focus solely on the wound itself. The end result of an holistic assessment should provide the nurse with a mosaic view of the patient that includes their general health, any underlying illnesses, psychological state and social circumstances, as well as their wound. This information can then be used to develop an individualised wound management programme. Such a programme should take into account not only the local wound environment but also the effect of the wound on the patient's psychological and social well being. In the case of chronic non-healing wounds, such as fungating lesions, where symptom control and improving or maintaining quality of life are paramount, this type of holistic assessment is vital (Laverty *et al.* 2000a).

3

Management of Specific Wound Types

Introduction

This chapter discusses the management of specific types of wounds. The characteristics of each wound are described, after which the management options available for that particular wound are outlined. To assist with cost-effectiveness, particular wound management products are recommended in the management options. Further information on these products is available in Chapter 5. A quick reference table for different wound types and symptoms is presented at the end of this chapter (Table 3.4). It must be remembered that any products mentioned should be used in accordance with the manufacturer's instructions.

NECROTIC WOUNDS

Definition

A necrotic wound contains tissue that has become devitalised due to damage to its blood supply, for example from pressure or trauma. When this tissue becomes dehydrated it forms a hard, black/brown leathery layer over the wound, commonly called an 'eschar' (Fig. 3.1) (Milward 1995, Cutting 1999).

Reference material

Eschar is composed of serous exudate, dead dermal cells, leucocytes and several extra-cellular components including collagen, fibrinogen and elastin (Thomas *et al.* 1999). As the necrotic tissue dries it contracts and may cause pain at the wound site (SMTL 1995). All devitalised tissue must be removed from the wound to prevent infection, promote granulation and allow assessment of the extent of tissue destruction (Bale 1997, Vowden & Vowden 1999a). Eschar needs to be detached from the wound base to allow epithelialisation, as epithelial cells cannot migrate over eschar (Milward 1995, Poston 1996). It should be noted that removal of an eschar often reveals a larger wound (Milward 1995).

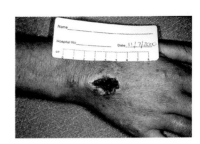

Fig. 3.1
Necrotic wound on the back of the hand
as a result of an extravasation injury.

Management options

Surgical debridement

This is the most rapid and effective method of debridement (Hampton 1999a).
It may be performed for extensive or deep areas of necrosis and often requires
a general anaesthetic in theatre. Only a skilled surgeon should perform surgical
debridement. The usefulness of this option must be balanced against the risk
to the patient from the general anaesthetic and the potential for damage to
underlying structures (Poston 1996, Vowden & Vowden 1999b, Werner 1999).

'Sharp' debridement

This method of debridement can be used to remove loose, devitalised, superficial tissue only. Sharp debridement should only be undertaken by health care
professionals who are competent in this method of debridement and after
consultation with the patient's medical team. It is usually performed at the
bedside using scissors and scalpel. A surgeon should perform debridement of
necrotic tissue that is deeper than the epidermal or dermal layers (Poston 1996,
Werner 1999).

Method of sharp debridement:
- Explain and discuss the procedure with the patient to ensure they understand
  the procedure.
- Position the patient comfortably and with the wound well exposed.
- Ensure the work area is well lit and large enough to allow easy movement
  around the patient.
- If the procedure will take a while consider having a chair to sit on beside the
  patient.

- Use aseptic technique (see also Hart 2000). Extra precautions, such as wearing a sterile gown, should be used for immunosuppressed patients.
- Use sterile instruments. These should include toothed forceps (easier to grip tissue with), scalpel handle and blade (size 10 or 15) and small, pointed, straight and/or curved scissors (iris scissors).
- Have extra low-linting gauze swabs, 0.9% sodium chloride, plastic aprons and sterile gloves available within the treatment area in case extra are needed during the procedure.
- Have an alginate dressing available in case of bleeding (for its haemostatic abilities).
- Wear a plastic apron and sterile gloves.
- Dissect devitalised tissue away slowly, always checking for, and avoiding, underlying structures.
- Only remove loose superficial tissue.
- After the procedure apply an appropriate dressing to the wound.

(Poston 1996, Bale 1997, Vowden & Vowden 1999b)

It may be useful to treat hard necrotic tissue with a hydrogel to soften the eschar (described below) prior to attempting sharp debridement. Repeated sessions may be necessary to remove all devitalised tissue.

Autolytic debridement

Autolysis is the body's natural debriding mechanism performed by neutrophils and macrophages. Maintaining a moist wound environment encourages this form of debridement (Hofman 1996, Bale 1997, Freedline 1999).

(1) Hydrogel

These dressings rehydrate eschar and promote autolysis of devitalised tissue (Bale 1997, Hampton 1999a, Werner 1999).

- Score the eschar with a scalpel to assist penetration of the gel.
- Apply gel directly to wound surface.
- Cover gel with an occlusive secondary dressing (for example a semi-permeable film dressing or hydrocolloid sheet).
- Leave undisturbed for 2–3 days, if possible, to allow adequate penetration of gel.
- Irrigate the wound at each dressing change to remove any loosened tissue.

- Use gel for (usually) at least 5 days to rehydrate and remove eschar.

(Gibson 1995, Hofman 1996, Williams 1996a, Bale 1997,
Thomas 1997, SMTL 1999)

(2) Hydrocolloid sheet
Retains moisture at the wound surface thereby promoting autolytic debridement.

- Apply hydrocolloid sheet directly to wound surface.
- Leave undisturbed for 2–3 days.
- Irrigate the wound at each dressing change to remove any loosened tissue.

(Thomas 1997, SMTL 1999)

Enzymatic debridement

Enzymes may be used in some circumstances where surgical debridement, particularly with a general anaesthetic, poses a risk to the patient and/or rehydration with a hydrogel has been ineffective. Use of the enzyme preparation Varidase® is described here:

- Reconstitute the enzyme with 5 ml of sterile water and add to 15 ml of a water-soluble medical lubricant (e.g. KY Jelly®).
- Apply directly to wound surface (score the eschar with a scalpel to assist penetration of the enzyme).

Alternatively:

- Reconstitute the enzyme with 20 ml of sterile 0.9% sodium chloride and cautiously inject below the eschar using a 25-gauge needle provided the patient can tolerate the increase in pressure produced by the fluid being injected under the eschar. This method should only be undertaken by competent practitioners.

With either method of enzyme application the following also applies:

- Cover the wound with an occlusive dressing to retain moisture (for example a semi-permeable film dressing or hydrocolloid sheet).
- Apply the enzyme once or twice daily.
- Irrigate the wound at each dressing change to remove any loosened tissue.
- Use until the eschar can be easily removed.

(Thomas 1990, Bennett & Moody 1995, Bale 1997)

Note: Gauze soaked in enzyme solution is not recommended as it dries very rapidly and may adhere to the wound, requires frequent changing and may cause maceration of surrounding skin (Thomas 1997).

Which management option?

There is relatively little supportive evidence for the use of any particular type of wound debridement (Bradley *et al.* 1999, Rodeheaver 1999). Therefore the method that is most appropriate for the patient should be used. The choice of management will depend on the position, type and depth of necrotic tissue as well as the patient's general health status (Werner 1999). For wounds with extensive or deep necrotic tissue, surgical or sharp debridement are usually the options of choice as they rapidly remove devitalised tissue thereby promoting the normal phases of wound healing and preventing infection (Werner 1999).

In certain cases surgical or sharp debridement should not be used: these include ischaemia due to arterial insufficiency, impaired blood clotting mechanism, malignant wounds and wounds with underlying structures close to the surface (Milward 1995, Poston 1996, Bale 1997, Hampton 1999a). When the patient's medical condition prevents surgical debridement or the tissue to be removed is not extensive and is superficial, then autolytic debridement is the option of choice. Enzymatic debridement is reserved for use if the autolytic method of debridement would take too long, or fails to adequately remove necrotic tissue (Freedline 1999, Werner 1999). It should be noted that there is evidence to suggest that the use of a hydrogel alone may be just as effective, and cheaper, than a mixture containing enzymes (Martin *et al.* 1996).

SLOUGHY WOUNDS

Definition

Slough refers to moist necrotic tissue. This type of devitalised tissue is soft, moist and often stringy in consistency and is usually yellow, white and/or grey in colour (Fig. 3.2) (Milward 1995, Poston 1996, Bale 1997).

Reference material

Slough has a similar composition to eschar tissue but has a larger number of leukocytes present and is moist. Slough must be removed to allow healing and to prevent colonisation and infection by microorganisms (Milward 1995, Bale

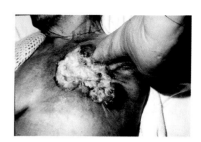

Fig. 3.2
A large amount of slough in a fungating
breast wound.

1997). Desloughing will usually take more than 3 days and it should be noted that wounds often increase in size as slough is removed; however this allows for better visualisation of the extent of the wound (Milward 1995).

Management options

The choice of management will depend on the position, type and depth of sloughy tissue as well as the patient's general health status (Werner 1999). Sloughy wounds often produce a large amount of exudate (Milward 1995), therefore management choice will depend largely on this aspect.

Surgical or sharp debridement

As described previously for necrotic wounds.

Autolytic debridement (see also necrotic wounds)

(1) Hydrogels

Hydrogels can be used provided there is none to moderate exudate. While the gels will absorb some exudate they cannot cope with high exudate levels.

- Apply gel directly to wound surface.
- Cover gel with an occlusive secondary dressing (for example a semi-permeable film dressing or hydrocolloid sheet).
- Leave undisturbed for 3 days, unless the dressing leaks, to allow for adequate action of the gel.
- If the wound is extremely sloughy, daily dressing changes may be required.
- Irrigate the wound at each dressing change to remove any loosened tissue.
  (Gibson 1995, Hofman 1996, Williams 1996a, Bale 1997, SMTL 1999)

51

The liquefaction of sloughy material may produce copious amounts of offensive appearing exudate. Patients should be informed of this possibility to prevent unnecessary anxiety (Poston 1996). If odour is a problem the hydrogel can be mixed with equal amounts of 0.8% metronidazole gel (Metrotop®) and applied to the wound. Daily dressing changes may also be required.

(2) Hydrocolloid sheets
Hydrocolloid sheets can also be used to maintain a moist wound environment (Milward 1995, Bale 1997, Thomas 1997).

- Apply sheet directly to wound with a 2–3 cm overlap from the wound margins.
- Leave dressing in place for 2–3 days if possible. The dressing may need to be changed more often if there is a large amount of exudate (consider using another type of dressing in this instance).
- Irrigate the wound at each dressing change to remove any loosened tissue.

(3) Foam cavity dressing + hydrogel
This is a useful combination for sloughy cavity wounds (Dunford 1997). However there is only a small amount of anecdotal evidence to support this combination (Stevens 1998, Thomas *et al*. 1998c). A hydrogel can be used to coat the foam plug to promote autolytic debridement of any sloughy areas on the cavity walls (Bale & Harding 1991, Young 1998).

- Select or prepare a foam dressing as appropriate and according to the relevant dressing information in Chapter 5.
- Cover the area of the foam dressing that will be in contact with the wound surface with the hydrogel.
- Place the prepared dressing into the cavity and secure with an appropriate secondary dressing.
- Irrigate the wound at each dressing change to remove any loosened tissue.

Enzymatic debridement
Enzymes are suitable for very thick sloughy areas. For best results the enzyme mixed with a water-soluble medical lubricant (e.g. KY Jelly®) should be used. Use of the enzyme preparation Varidase® is described below.

- Reconstitute the enzyme with 5 ml of sterile water and add to 15 ml of a water-soluble medical lubricant (e.g. KY Jelly®).
- Apply directly to wound surface.
- Cover with an occlusive dressing to retain moisture (for example a semi-permeable film dressing or hydrocolloid sheet).
- Apply enzyme once to twice daily.
- Irrigate the wound at each dressing change to remove any loosened tissue.
- Use until the slough can be easily removed.

(Morison 1992, Bennett & Moody 1995, Bale 1997)

Larval therapy

This involves the use of fly larvae (maggots) to remove sloughy/necrotic tissue. This therapy is also useful for treating recalcitrant infections or antibiotic-resistant bacteria such as MRSA (Thomas *et al.* 1999a).

- Trace the wound onto a plastic sheet and transfer the wound shape to a hydro-colloid sheet. It is best to use a large sheet and cut an area out of the middle.
- Surround the wound with the hydrocolloid sheet to protect the skin from enzymes produced by the larvae and to prevent the escape of any maggots. A zinc paste bandage can be used on fragile skin in place of the hydrocolloid if necessary.
- Using sterile 0.9% sodium chloride, wash the larvae out of the transport bottle onto a piece of nylon net (usually supplied), which in turn should be resting upon a dressing pad to absorb excess fluid.
- Apply the larvae to the wound using the nylon net as a cover to keep the larvae in place. It is recommended that a maximum of 10 larvae be applied per cm^2 of wound surface.
- Secure the nylon net in place by taping it to the hydrocolloid sheet (a water-resistant tape such as Sleek® is suggested) or pressing it into the zinc bandage.
- Cover the nylon net with a dressing pad (e.g. Surgipad®) moistened with sterile 0.9% sodium chloride.
- Place a secondary absorbent pad over this and hold it in place with a bandage. *Note:* Occlusive dressings should not be used, as the larvae need to breathe.
- Leave the larvae in place for up to 3 days but change the outer pad daily or as necessary. The degradation of slough will produce more exudate, which may also have an offensive odour.

Shallow wound with low exudate

(1) Hydrocolloid sheet
- Apply directly to wound surface.
- Change every 3–5 days (may be left for up to 7 days in low exudate wounds).

(2) Hydrogel sheet
- Apply directly to wound surface.
- Change every 2–3 days.
- May be re-hydrated *in situ* by irrigating with 0.9% sodium chloride.

(3) Hydrogel
- Apply directly to wound surface.
- Cover with an occlusive dressing.
- Change every 2–3 days.

(4) Semi-permeable film dressings
- Apply directly to wound surface.
- Change every 2–3 days.

Shallow wound with high exudate

(1) Alginate sheet
- Apply directly to wound surface.
- Cover with a secondary dressing as appropriate.
- Change when strike-through occurs (or at least twice weekly).

(2) Hydrofibre sheet
- Apply directly to wound surface.
- Cover with a secondary dressing as appropriate.
- Change when strike-through occurs (or at least twice weekly).

(3) Foam sheets
- Apply directly to wound surface.
- Secure with hypoallergenic tape or tubular net bandage (if the foam is self-adhesive this should be unnecessary).
- Change when strike-through occurs (or at least weekly).

Deep wound with low exudate

(1) Hydrogel
- Apply directly to wound surface.
- Cover with an occlusive dressing (for example a semi-permeable film dressing or hydrocolloid sheet).
- Change every 2–3 days.

(2) Silicone polymer foam cavity dressing
- Prepare the dressing (Cavi-Care®) to the manufacturer's instructions.
- Insert the dressing into the wound.
- Secure with hypoallergenic tape.
- Remove the dressing and wash it (according to the manufacturer's instructions) at least once every 48 hours.

Deep wound with high exudate

(1) Alginate ribbon or packing
- Apply directly to wound surface.
- Cover with a secondary dressing as appropriate.
- Change when strike-through occurs.

(2) Hydrofibre ribbon
- Apply directly to wound surface.
- Cover with a secondary dressing as appropriate.
- Change when strike-through occurs.

(3) Polyurethane foam cavity dressing
- Insert the dressing into the wound.
- Cover with a secondary absorbent dressing.
- Secure with hypoallergenic tape.
- Change when strike-through occurs.
- Allevyn Cavity® dressing is suggested.

(Miller & Dyson 1996, Morgan 1997, Hampton 1999a)

Appropriate secondary dressings include absorbent pads and foam sheets.

Which management option?

The choice of management will depend on the depth of the wound and the amount of exudate being produced, as well as the need to maintain a moist wound environment. For wounds with a high amount of exudate a dressing product with an ability to absorb excess exudate, while maintaining a moist wound environment, should be used. This will prevent exudate leakage and thus maceration of surrounding skin (Bale & Jones 1997). For wounds with low levels of exudate a less absorbent dressing is recommended as it will not remove all of the exudate, thereby maintaining a moist wound bed. This prevents the wound from drying out and the dressing adhering to the wound. Newly epithelialising wounds generally do not produce much exudate but require protection of the delicate new epithelium. Also, a moist wound environment will encourage migration of epithelial cells (Miller & Dyson 1996). These conditions are most commonly achieved by applying a semi-permeable film or thin hydrocolloid sheet over the wound and then for a further 5–7 days after complete epithelialisation (Morison 1992). Choosing a dressing that can remain in place for a number of days (e.g. a hydrocolloid) is also beneficial as disturbing the wound with unnecessary dressing changes could damage granulating or epithelialising tissues and delay healing (Morison 1992, Flanagan 1998).

INFECTED WOUNDS

Definition

An infected wound is one that has been colonised by pathogenic bacteria and in which a host reaction has been initiated (Cutting 1998, Gilchrist 1999).

Reference material

The presence of bacteria in a wound does not necessarily indicate an infection or the need for antibiotics (Cutting 1998, Miller 1998b). Wounds are not sterile and many chronic wounds will heal in the presence of bacterial colonisation (Fletcher 1997, Miller 1998b). It is generally agreed that clinical infection occurs at greater than or equal to 10^5 bacteria per gram of tissue, although this level may not apply to all patients. In particular immunosuppressed patients may show signs of clinical infection at a much lower level (Cutting 1998, Miller 1998b). Signs and symptoms of clinical infection (Table 3.1) manifest at the

Table 3.1
Signs and symptoms of
wound infection.

(1) Erythema (redness and heat)
(2) Pain
(3) Oedema
(4) Heavy exudate
(5) Malodour
(6) Generalised pyrexia

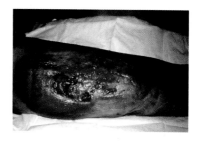

Fig. 3.5
An infected venous leg ulcer showing
signs of erythema and oedema as well as
unhealthy granulation tissue. The wound
was also painful and malodorous
(photograph kindly supplied by Johnson &
Johnson Medical).

wound site and/or surrounding tissues (Fig. 3.5) (Miller & Dyson 1996, Miller 1998b, Gilchrist 1999).

Care needs to be taken with patients who are immunosuppressed, on systemic steroid therapy or who have a chronic wound. These patients will often not display the characteristic signs and symptoms of clinical infection (Cutting 1998, Gilchrist 1999). For these patients, clinical infection may present as deterioration of the wound (Table 3.2). The risk of a patient acquiring a wound infection is influenced by a number of factors (Table 3.3).

The Public Health Laboratory Service undertook a national nosocomial infection surveillance scheme, which reviewed surgical wound infections in 70 English hospitals. Of the types of surgical operations included in this study, infection rates varied from 1.8% for abdominal hysterectomy surgery, to 15.2% for gastric surgery. Whilst most of the infections were superficial, for small and large bowel surgery 40% of these infections were more serious. The microorganisms that were the most common cause of infection were staphylococci, of which 80% were *Staphylococcus aureus*, 67% of which were Methicillin resistant (i.e. MRSA) (PHLS 1999).

When a wound infection is suspected, based on the signs and symptoms in Tables 3.1 and 3.2, a microbiology swab of the wound should be taken. It is

Table 3.2 Signs and symptoms of infection in chronic wounds.

(1) Delayed healing
(2) Breakdown of wound
(3) Presence of friable granulation tissue that bleeds easily
(4) Formation of an epithelial tissue bridge over the wound
(5) Increased production of exudate and malodour
(6) Increased pain

(Miller & Dyson 1996, Cutting 1998, Miller 1998b, Gilchrist 1999)

Table 3.3 Factors that influence wound infection.

Main factors	Secondary factors
(1) Immune status of the patient	(1) Duration of surgery
(2) Underlying disease	(2) Presence of devitalised tissue
(3) Nutritional status	(3) Tissue damage during procedure
(4) Length of pre-operative stay in hospital	(4) Haematoma formation
(5) Pre-operative preparation	(5) Presence of foreign material
(6) Obesity	(6) The presence, number and virulence of pathogenic microorganisms
(7) Older age	

(Cruse & Ford 1980, Kernoble & Kaiser 1995, Wilson 1995, Bertin *et al.* 1998, Moore & Foster 1998a)

best taken before cleaning the wound when the maximum number of organisms will be present. Swab containers should contain special transport medium, which will help to preserve the microorganisms during transit to the microbiology department. Swabs must be clearly labelled and the request card must state the exact site from which the swab was obtained and which, if any, antibiotics the patient is currently taking.

The need for the patient with an infected wound to receive systemic antibiotics will depend on whether the signs and symptoms of infection are increasing, and on the general immune status of the patient. However, it is recommended that once a diagnosis of clinical infection has been reached, systemic antibiotic treatment should be commenced (Morison 1992, Miller 1998b). Antibiotic therapy should be guided by the results of the microbiology swab of the wound, although it cannot be guaranteed that the swab will isolate the infecting organism (Gilchrist 1999).

Management options

Cleansing solutions

It is generally agreed that warmed, sterile, 0.9% sodium chloride is the best irrigating solution and all that is necessary for the cleansing of infected wounds (Miller & Dyson 1996, Fletcher 1997, Gilchrist 1999). Tap water may be used to soak off large dressings. A number of authors have recommended using tap water to cleanse chronic wounds such as leg ulcers (Fletcher 1997, Gilchrist 1999). However, cleansing wounds with tap water is not recommended for patients with compromised immunity because of their increased susceptibility to infection.

Dressing choice

The following dressings may be used on infected wounds. Dressing selection will depend upon the wound type, size and amount of exudate.

Shallow wound with low exudate

(1) Hydrocolloid sheet
- Apply directly to wound surface.
- Change daily (note that this may not be cost-effective).

(2) Hydrogel sheet
- Apply directly to wound surface.
- Change daily.
- May be re-hydrated *in situ* by irrigating with 0.9% sodium chloride.

Note: Some hydrogel sheets are contraindicated for *Pseudomonas aeruginosa* infections (e.g. Geliperm®).

Shallow wound with high exudate

(1) Alginate sheet
- Apply directly to wound surface.
- Cover with a secondary dressing as appropriate.
- Change daily.

(2) Hydrofibre sheet
- Apply directly to wound surface.
- Cover with a secondary dressing as appropriate.
- Change daily.

(3) Foam sheets
- Apply directly to wound surface.
- Secure with hypoallergenic tape or tubular net bandage (if the foam is self-adhesive this should be unnecessary).
- Change daily.

Deep wound with low exudate

(1) Hydrogel
- Apply directly to wound surface.
- Cover with an occlusive dressing (for example a semi-permeable film dressing or hydrocolloid sheet).
- Change daily.

(2) Silicone polymer foam cavity dressing
- *Prepare the dressing (Cavi-Care®) according to the manufacturer's instructions.*
- Insert the dressing into the wound.
- Secure with hypoallergenic tape.
- Remove the dressing and wash it (according to the manufacturer's instructions) at least once every 24 hours (as opposed to every 48 hours for clean wounds).

Deep wound with high exudate

(1) Alginate ribbon or packing
- Apply directly to wound surface.
- Cover with a secondary dressing as appropriate.
- Change daily.

(2) Hydrofibre ribbon
- Apply directly to wound surface.
- Cover with a secondary dressing as appropriate.
- Change daily.

(3) Polyurethane foam cavity dressing
- Insert the dressing to the wound.
- Cover with a secondary absorbent dressing.
- Secure with hypoallergenic tape.
- Change daily.
- Allevyn Cavity® is suggested.

(Thomas 1994, Miller & Dyson 1996)

Appropriate secondary dressings include absorbent pads and foam sheets.

Which management option?

Dressing choice depends primarily on the size of the wound and the amount of exudate being produced. If the patient is infected with a communicable disease or an organism with multiple antibiotic resistance they may need to be barrier nursed (using the source isolation technique) to control the spread of the organism (Hart 2000). An occlusive dressing may also be employed to prevent the spread of the organism (Thomas 1997).

Ensure that the patient is aware of their wound infection, particularly if it is communicable, and also the type of treatment, if any, they are receiving. The risk of wound infection and cross infection is reduced by the use of an aseptic technique whilst changing wound dressings (Briggs *et al.* 1996). Hand washing is essential both before and after wound care (if hands are contaminated during the procedure they should be cleaned with an alcohol handrub), along with careful disposal of used dressings and lotions. In addition, dressings, tape and equipment must not be shared between patients.

CAVITY WOUNDS

Definition

A cavity is a 'hollow area' created due to a degree of tissue loss (Fig. 3.6) (Bale & Collier 1998). The cavity may be shallow or deep and may be due to surgical

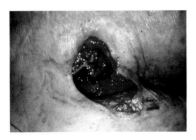

Fig. 3.6
A full thickness sacral pressure ulcer with a deep cavity and undermining of the surrounding skin (photograph kindly supplied by Johnson & Johnson Medical).

debridement, trauma, breakdown of tissue due to pressure or disease, or dehiscence of a surgical wound (Hallett 1995a).

Reference material

The aim of cavity wound care is to promote formation of granulation tissue from the base of the wound upwards. Pressure on the wound bed can initiate formation of granulation tissue but if the cavity is packed too tightly, for example with ribbon gauze, this will cause shearing and damage to the new tissue (Dawson *et al*. 1992). Cavity wounds will undergo many changes in shape and therefore frequent reassessment is required to select the correct product depending on the presenting symptoms and shape/depth of the wound.

Management options

Traditionally ribbon gauze soaked in antiseptic solutions, in particular Proflavine®, was used to pack a cavity wound. This practice is now considered to be unsuitable. It causes pain for the patient, needs to be changed frequently to prevent adherence to the wound bed, and granulation tissue can grow into the gauze and be damaged or removed when the dressing is changed (Dawson *et al*. 1992, Berry & Jones 1993).

Low exudate

(1) Hydrogel
- Apply directly to wound surface.
- Cover with an occlusive dressing (for example a semi-permeable film dressing or hydrocolloid sheet).
- Change every 2–3 days.

(2) Silicone polymer foam cavity dressing
- Prepare the dressing (Cavi-Care®) according to the manufacturer's instructions.
- Insert the dressing into the wound.
- Secure with hypoallergenic tape.
- Remove the dressing and wash it (according to the manufacturer's instructions) at least once every 48 hours.

High exudate

(1) Hydrofibre ribbon or Alginate ribbon or packing
- Lightly pack into the wound.
- Cover with a secondary absorbent dressing as appropriate (for example an absorbent pad or foam sheet dressing).
- Change when strike-through occurs.

(2) Polyurethane foam cavity dressings
- Carefully insert the dressing into the wound.
- Cover with a secondary absorbent dressing, as appropriate.
- Secure with hypoallergenic tape.
- Change when strike-through occurs.
- Allevyn Cavity® is suggested.

(Miller & Dyson 1996, Morgan 1997, Hampton 1999a)

Which management option?

The choice of management will depend on the size of the cavity and the type of tissue present. The volume of exudate being produced will also need to be taken into account. After assessing the wound, refer to the appropriate wound type, e.g. necrotic, sloughy, granulating or infected, for further guidance on wound management options.

SINUS WOUNDS

Definition

A sinus wound is an abnormal, blind-ended tract leading from the skin or wound surface into the body tissues (Fig. 3.7) (Morison 1992, Bennett & Moody 1995).

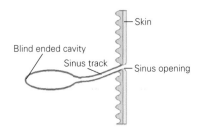

Fig. 3.7
A sinus (© Wayne Naylor 2000).

The origin of the sinus may be a cavity, which has the potential to become a focus of infection, or an abscess (Dealey 1999).

Reference material

Ideally, the aim is to prevent a sinus forming by keeping the wound edges apart and encouraging healing of the wound from the base. It is important to prevent 'bridges' of granulation tissue or skin forming along the length of the sinus. This may result in the formation of a 'dead space' underneath the surface of the skin, which could predispose to infection. A probe can be gently used to investigate the depth and size of the sinus, especially if it is unclear where the sinus originates.

Management options

The most effective way to manage a sinus is to lay it open by surgical intervention. However, allowing the area to discharge freely through a drainage tube may be a more appropriate option if the sinus is very deep and narrow. The tube can be gradually withdrawn as the sinus heals (Everett 1985). Care should be taken to avoid putting any wound management product into the sinus that could easily separate and leave particulate matter in the wound on removal, such as cotton wool. Retention of any foreign material will add to the potential risk of infection. The following products may be indicated for use in sinus management depending on the presenting symptoms:

(1) Silicone polymer foam cavity dressing
- Prepare the stent according to the manufacturer's instructions (see Chapter 5).
- Insert the stent into the wound.

- Apply a secondary absorbent dressing if necessary.
- Secure with hypoallergenic tape.

(2) Hydrofibre ribbon or Alginate ribbon
- Carefully insert the ribbon into the sinus using a probe to ensure that the dressing reaches as far into the sinus as possible, but do not pack too tightly.
- Cover with a secondary absorbent dressing.
- Secure with hypoallergenic tape.

(3) Honey or thin sugar paste
- Draw the honey or sugar paste into a syringe.
- Carefully fill the sinus from the syringe.
- Cover with a secondary absorbent dressing.
- Secure with hypoallergenic tape.

Which management option?

The choice of management will depend on the size and depth of the sinus and how much exudate it is producing. For copious amounts of exudate a highly absorbent dressing should be used, such as a hydrofibre. For an infected sinus honey or sugar paste may be useful due to their antibacterial properties (Morgan 1997, Molan 1999d). The silicone polymer foam stent should not be used in deep narrow sinuses due to the possibility of small pieces breaking off and remaining in the wound (SMTL 1999).

FISTULAE

Definition

Fistulae are abnormal openings between two epithelial lined surfaces. They may be external, running between hollow viscera and the skin, or internal, connecting two hollow viscera without communication to the body surface (Martin 1996).

Reference material

Fistulae that connect the gastrointestinal system and the skin are referred to as enterocutaneous fistulae. They occur most commonly after bowel surgery and usually as the result of sepsis, an insubstantial anastomosis or a distal obstruc-

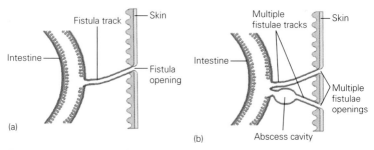

Fig. 3.8 (a) A simple fistula (© Wayne Naylor 2000). (b) A complex fistula (© Wayne Naylor 2000).

tion. They are also associated with inflammatory bowel disease, diverticular disease, malignancy, trauma and radiotherapy (Bennett & Moody 1995, Forbes & Myers 1996, Meadows 1997). Fistulae may be simple (Fig. 3.8a), multiple or complicated (Fig. 3.8b) and any of these may also be obstructed. A simple unobstructed fistula is likely to heal with supportive care, whereas a complex fistula (for example where two ends of bowel communicate via an abscess cavity) will require surgical intervention.

Aims of management

Management of enterocutaneous fistulae is dependent on the fistula characteristics. The aim of fistula management should incorporate the following principles:

- Protection of surrounding skin.
- Collection and containment of fistula output.
- Control of odour.
- Promotion of confidence and a sense of well being.

Assessment

Assessment of the fistula site and the type of effluent drainage are important for successful management. Fistula sites may be classified using the following descriptive categories:

- *Grade 1*   The fistula has a single orifice passing through an intact abdominal wall or otherwise healed scar, surrounded by flat intact skin.

- *Grade 2*   The fistula has a single/multiple orifice(s) passing through the abdominal wall close to a bony prominence, surgical scar, stoma or the umbilicus.
- *Grade 3*   The fistula has an orifice situated in a small dehiscence of the abdominal wall.
- *Grade 4*   The fistula has an orifice situated in a large dehiscence of the abdominal wall or within a gaping wound.

(Irving & Beadle 1982)

Fistulae may be further classified by the amount of effluent drainage. Less than 500 ml in 24 hours is described as low-output, while greater than 500 ml in 24 hours is described as high-output. Areas of reddened and broken skin surrounding the fistula should also be noted as they may be the cause of pain or discomfort and can impede the adherence of an appliance.

The volume, consistency and type of effluent draining will influence the aids and appliances required for the management of the fistula. For example, a high-output fistula will need a secondary drainage system. For thin, or watery, effluent a urostomy pouch attached to a catheter bag will be sufficient but if the effluent is thicker the appliances used should have a wide bore outlet or an access window (for example the ConvaTec® Wound Manager™). The access window allows for the appliance to be flushed out as necessary to keep the pouch clean and reduce odour.

Drainage from fistulae in the upper gastrointestinal tract contains proteolytic secretions that will digest skin, causing excoriation, ulceration, infection and pain. These secretions will also quickly reduce the effectiveness of appliances and adhesives. Therefore appliances may need to be changed more regularly and any leaks must not be 'patched up' (Forbes & Myers 1996, Meadows 1997).

Management options

Skin excoriation

(1) Skin barrier films
- Protect the skin from excoriation by proteolytic secretions.
- Prevent skin stripping by adhesives.
- Use alcohol-free products that will not cause stinging if applied to broken areas of skin (see Chapter 5 for more information on skin barrier films).

(2) Pastes (for example Stomahesive Paste^{TM})

- Use to fill creases, crevices or gullies in the skin to provide a smooth surface for the application of a stoma or wound management appliance.
- Do not use on unprotected broken skin as these products contain alcohol and will cause pain and stinging.
- May be piped into creases using a syringe.
- Leave to dry for 60 s or dry with a warm hairdryer after application to the skin.
- Mould and pat the paste into the skin crease.
- Before moulding, wet fingers with water to prevent the paste from sticking to fingers.

(3) Protective pastes (for example Orabase Paste^{TM})

- Designed to protect mucous membranes and skin.
- Similar in composition to Stomahesive Paste^{TM} but with the addition of liquid paraffin, therefore will prevent any adhesives from sticking.
- Apply to the skin between small fistula orifices or may be applied to the edges of cavities or large fistulae.
- Reapply as necessary if the appliance used has an access window.

(4) Powders (for example Orahesive Powder^{TM})

- Use for the protection of sore or raw areas without impeding the adhesion of appliances.
- May also be used on raw areas to form a protective layer before applying paste.
- Apply sparingly and dust off excess or the extra powder may impede adhesion of the appliance.

(5) Cohesive washers (for example Salts Cohesive Seals®)

- Use to provide skin protection around fistula.
- May be used to fill in creases or gullies.

(6) Hydrocolloid wafers (for example Duoderm®, Comfeel^{TM} Wafer, Stomahesive^{TM} Wafer)

- Use to protect skin from proteolytic secretions.
- Use to provide an even flat surface on areas where paste has been used to fill in creases, crevices or gullies prior to application of appliance.

Table 3.4 Wound management products for specific wound types and symptoms.

| | Wound management products for specific symptoms | | | |
| | Deep cavity | | Shallow wound | |
Description of wound	low exudate	high exudate	low exudate	high exudate
Necrotic Hard tissue that is brown or black in colour (leathery appearance). Should be removed to allow granulation and prevent infection	Requires debridement by: Surgery/sharp debridement Hydrogel/hydrocolloid gel Enzymes (use with caution)			
Sloughy Soft, moist and stringy tissue that is yellow, white and/or grey in colour. Needs to be removed to allow granulation and prevent infection. Enzymes or larval therapy can be used if other methods fail	Hydrogel +/− foam cavity dressing	Alginate/ hydrofibre VAC therapy	Hydrogel Hydrocolloid sheet	Alginate/ hydrofibre VAC therapy
Granulating Pink/red granular tissue, which may bleed easily Requires protection Do not change dressing frequently	Hydrogel Foam cavity dressing	Alginate/ hydrofibre Foam cavity dressing	Hydrogel sheet/gel Hydrocolloid sheet Semi-permeable film	Alginate/ hydrofibre Foam sheet
Epithelialising Pink/white tissue, still fragile Requires protection	Thin hydrocolloid sheet Hydrogel sheet Semi-permeable film			
Infected Identified by clinical signs: pain, heat, swelling and redness +/− purulent discharge. May require systemic antibiotic. Irrigate with 0.9% sodium chloride – do not use topical antiseptics/ antibiotics. Dressing should be changing daily	Hydrogel Foam cavity dressing	Alginate/ hydrofibre Foam cavity dressing	Hydrogel sheet Hydrocolloid sheet	Alginate/ hydrofibre Foam sheet
Malodorous Need to remove slough and necrotic tissue Eradicate organisms causing odour Can use dressings to absorb odour	Metronidazole gel (plus hydrocolloid gel for sloughy/necrotic wounds) Honey/sugar paste + secondary dressing of choice +/− activated charcoal dressing			

Appliances/dressings

There are numerous appliances that may be used in fistula management. For example, large postoperative stoma pouches, high-output stoma pouches, wound managers, fistula pouches and paediatric ostomy appliances are all possibilities. The most appropriate device will depend on the size, shape and site of the fistula as well as the volume, consistency and type of effluent draining.

Dressings may be used in conjunction with appliances, for example packing and covering part of a wound above a high-output area can make it easier to contain the discharge with a smaller pouch.

If managed appropriately most fistulae will heal spontaneously; however for a small number of patients a fistula may become a chronic problem, especially if it is associated with an inflammatory condition or malignancy (Bennett & Moody 1995). Surgical intervention to excise the fistula may be necessary in these instances (Dealey 1999). Particular attention needs to be paid to the maintenance of intact skin and containment of effluent to allow the patient to live as free a life as possible. Patients with high-output stomas may also need dietary advice as they can suffer from malnutrition and dehydration related to the loss of body fluids.

CONCLUSION

This chapter has presented the management of wounds according to their appearance or symptoms. The management options outlined may be used for any wound following an in-depth assessment (Table 3.4). If a wound has multiple symptoms or consists of more than one type of tissue, then management options may be combined to treat all aspects of the wound. While most wounds, whether complex or chronic, can be managed according to their symptoms and/or appearance, it must be remembered that the underlying cause of the wound will have to be addressed when developing a wound management care plan. For example, cancer patients may develop wounds that are related to their disease or treatment. These wounds commonly have unusual or complex characteristics and often require specialised care. The next chapter discusses these wounds and outlines particular management strategies.

4

Management of Wounds Related to Cancer and Cancer Therapies

Introduction

The cells of a malignant tumour do not behave in a coherent or orderly way. They can invade local tissues and organs or spread to distant sites in the body (metastasis) (Weinberg 1996). Therefore the treatment of cancer is often intense and highly invasive in order to remove or destroy all of the tumour cells present in the body. Due to the intensity of the treatments employed to fight cancer, patients often have significant side effects. Often, these treatments can result in the formation of wounds that may, in some cases, be simple to manage but are more often complex and require a well-planned management strategy. Cancer itself can give rise to wounds in the form of skin lesions or 'fungating' wounds. These wounds frequently have multiple associated symptoms and can be difficult for the patient and their family to come to terms with. This chapter highlights the different types of wounds that may be associated with cancer or its treatment and offers guidance on their management.

SURGICAL WOUNDS

Definition

A surgical wound is a wound created during a surgical procedure to access structures or organs underlying the skin, remove diseased tissue or repair a traumatic injury (Moore & Foster 1998a).

Reference material

Surgical wounds are most commonly repaired by bringing the tissue edges together with sutures, clips or adhesive strips. Drains may be placed in the wound bed to prevent the formation of collections of serous fluid (seroma) or blood (haematoma) (Moore & Foster 1998a). Sutured wounds have no visible granulation tissue and generally heal with minimal scar formation (primary intention healing) (Collier 1996, Miller & Dyson 1996). Some surgical wounds may be left open to heal by secondary intention, for example an abscess or wide local excision of a tumour (Collier 1996, Miller & Dyson 1996, Moore & Foster 1998a). In some instances delayed primary intention healing may be indicated for surgical wounds that are contaminated or infected.

Management options

Open wounds

These wounds will heal by secondary or delayed primary intention (Fig. 4.1). After assessing the wound's appearance, refer to the appropriate section in Chapter 3 concerning management (i.e. necrotic, sloughy, granulating and epithelialising or infected) or the quick reference guide (Table 3.4).

Closed wounds

For sutured wounds (Fig. 4.2) a dressing that protects the wound from external contamination, and prevents soiling of the patient's clothing, is usually all that is necessary. The two dressings most commonly used are adhesive island dressings and semi-permeable films.

(1) Adhesive island dressing
- Apply dressing directly to clean suture line.
- May be removed 24–48 hours post operatively.

(Foster & Moore 1998, SMTL 1999)

(2) Semi-permeable film dressing
- Apply dressing directly to clean suture line.
- May be removed 24–48 hours postoperatively.

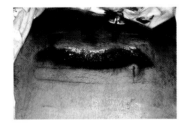

Fig. 4.1
A healing laparotomy wound left open following complications of major gastrointestinal surgery.

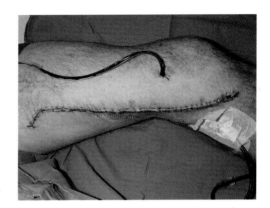

Fig. 4.2
A surgical wound closed
with staples following
excision of a sarcoma
from the leg.

- Can be left in place for several days (maximum 7 days).
- Patients may bathe with the dressing in place.

(Foster & Moore 1998, SMTL 1999)

Which management option?

Adhesive island dressings are useful for lightly exuding suture lines. Semi-permeable film dressings allow for observation of the wound, as they are transparent, but they cannot absorb exudate. However, if fluid does accumulate under the dressing it can be aspirated using a needle and syringe (Miller & Dyson 1996, SMTL 1999). Surgical wound dressings are usually removed 48 hours postoperatively and the wound left exposed. However, if the sight of the wound is distressing to the patient, or they experience discomfort from clothing rubbing on the wound, it may be necessary to continue to apply dressings to the wound (Galvani 1997). A surgical wound dressing over a suture line should be changed if it becomes stained by discharge or if the patient displays clinical signs of infection, either generalised or locally at the wound site (see section on infected wounds in Chapter 3) (Bale & Jones 1997).

PLASTIC SURGERY WOUNDS

Definition

Plastic surgery wounds are the result of surgical techniques, using flaps and skin grafts, for the purpose of reconstruction (remoulding and reshaping of tissues), including restoration of function and cosmetic appearance (Brown *et al.* 1998).

Reference material

Plastic surgery is frequently utilised following the excision of malignant or benign tumours, and for the repair of congenital abnormalities or traumatic injuries (including burns). The nursing care of these wounds relies on the development of specialist nursing skills. However, the fundamentals of nursing care should not be forgotten. Wound care for these patients, as with all wounds, requires an individualised approach and is dependent on many factors. These include the amount of exudate, presence of infection and the type of wound. In addition to these major factors the anatomical site of the wound must be considered, for example intra-oral, upper arm or breast. Overall, easy access to the wound is of paramount importance in order to assess the wound and to evaluate the effectiveness and patient comfort of dressings and securing materials.

For the patient undergoing plastic surgery the process from initial consultation with the plastic surgeon through to rehabilitation is often lengthy. However, this ensures that the patient has sufficient preoperative explanation and also sufficient time to discuss the impact of surgery, not only with health care professionals but also with a partner, friends or family. The patient's ability to adjust to the resulting changes in body image, function and cosmesis, and to reintegrate into society will vary from individual to individual (Fig. 4.3). Regular assessment is therefore crucial, enabling the plastic surgeon, nurses and other members of the multi-professional team (e.g. physiotherapist and speech and language therapist) to assess the patient's progress. Over time, as the wound healing process continues, the plastic surgeon is able to assess and discuss with the patient any need for further intervention, for example further surgery, which may be required to improve function or aesthetics. The support of these patients is therefore an integral part of the nurse's role and requires a collaborative approach between hospital and community nurses.

Surgical flaps

A surgical flap is an area of tissue that is transferred from one anatomical site to another with a functioning blood supply (Coull 1992, Brown *et al.* 1998), which is used for the purpose of reconstructing a defect. A flap usually consists of

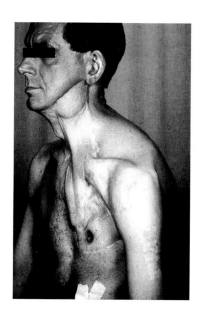

Fig. 4.3
Cosmetic result of a healed delto-pectoral flap used to reconstruct the neck. Consent for publication kindly given by the patient.

skin plus several layers of underlying tissues, which may include fat, fascia, and muscle or bone (Coull 1992). A flap may be used to restore function and cosmetic appearance, to enhance or increase vascularity or to cover important exposed structures such as tendons, blood vessels, nerves and bones (Clamon & Netscher 1994). The main aim of wound care in this instance is to ensure that the flap remains viable (healthy).

Types of flaps

Flaps can be moved from a location immediately adjacent to the defect (local flap) or from a site distant from the defect (Clamon & Netscher 1994). Either type is reliant on a functioning blood supply and this can be obtained by using one of two ways of transferring tissue – a 'free flap' or a 'pedicled flap'. A free flap is completely detached from the donor area along with its arterial and venous blood vessels. Using microvascular surgery techniques, these vessels are then reattached to blood vessels at the recipient site (Brown *et al.* 1998). Plastic and reconstructive surgeons are reliant on the microscope and micro-instruments to anastomose (artificially connect) blood vessels and nerves that may be less than 2 mm in diameter (Westlake 1991).

A pedicled flap (Fig. 4.4) remains attached to its original blood supply and is rotated or tunnelled into the new position (Rodzwic & Donnard 1986). The stem that contains the blood vessels (and possibly nerves) and attaches the flap to its original donor site is called a pedicle. This may also be known as a 'regional flap' as the flap is still attached to the region from where it originates. Flaps can also be classified according to their blood supply, the type of tissue involved, the method by which they reach the defect and their distance from the defect (Clamon & Netscher 1994).

The overall aims when using a flap to reconstruct a defect are to use a flap which:

(1) Has appropriate bulk or level of thickness in order to fill the cavity and restore function and cosmetic appearance.
(2) Is similar in colour and texture to the recipient site in order to provide camouflage and act in a similar physiological way as surrounding tissue.

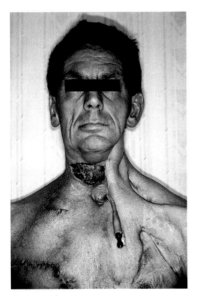

Fig. 4.4
A pedicled latissimus dorsi flap used to repair a fistula in the anterior neck. Note that the pedicle can be seen running under the skin diagonally across the right side of the chest. Consent for publication kindly given by the patient.

(3) Is as anatomically near, or adjacent, to the recipient site as is feasibly possible, thereby minimising any potential complications.

(4) Enables its donor site to be repaired with the minimum of further disfigurement and dysfunction.

A flap should be chosen that has the least potential donor morbidity and yet achieves the reconstructive demands (Clamon & Netscher 1994).

Classification of flaps

There are three main types of flaps, classified according to their blood supply and the type of tissue involved – random pattern flaps, axial pattern flaps and myocutaneous flaps.

Random pattern flaps

These, as the name suggests, have a random pattern of blood vessels. There is no clearly defined artery or vein running in the long axis of the flap (Coull 1992). The skin in these flaps survives on blood vessels from the subdermal skin plexus, which provides a blood supply many times in excess of the metabolic requirements of the skin. This is because of the skins important role in regulating temperature (Davies 1985b).

The flap remains attached to a pedicle on one side, which contains the nerves and blood vessels which keep the flap viable (Edwards 1994). This flap is therefore suitable only to be used as a local flap where the skin next to the defect is used, for example the excision of a basal cell carcinoma of the cheek, which is repaired using adjacent skin. There are four types of local flaps:

(1) *Rotation flap* – The skin and fat are rotated around a pivot point to cover an adjacent defect (Edwards 1994).

(2) *Transposition flap* – The flap is rotated across and over a defect, resulting in a deficit at the original flap donor site. This requires closure with a skin graft or with suturing.

(3) *Rhomboid flap* – This has a sloping rectangular shape (Edwards 1994) and enables a lesion to be excised in the rhomboid shape, then closed using sutures.

(4) *Advancement flap* – These flaps do not require rotation to fill a defect but are gently stretched, to 'advance' the flap to cover the defect.

Axial pattern flaps

This flap has an anatomically recognised artery and vein running in its long axis. For example skin on the anterior chest wall may be raised as a long flap, known as the deltopectoral flap, based on perforating branches from the internal mammary artery (Davies 1985b). This flap is often used for pharyngeal reconstruction following a partial pharyngectomy. On specific areas of the body much longer flaps can be raised because the flap has a specific anatomical blood vessel in its pedicle (Davies 1985b).

Myocutaneous flaps

These consist of a muscle, with the overlying skin, and have an anatomically recognised artery and vein (Edwards 1994). Large areas of skin are not supplied on an axial basis but are supplied by perforating vessels coming through from underlying muscles (Davies 1985b). Muscles usually receive their blood supply via vessels at one end, therefore the other end of the muscle may be detached and the muscle isolated on a pedicle with or without the overlying skin (Davies 1985b).

Management of flaps

Regular observation, particularly of free flaps, is essential (Coull 1992). Pedicled flaps should also be closely monitored as the pedicle can become twisted impairing circulation and resulting in flap necrosis. To determine the frequency of flap observations the nurse should liaise with the plastic surgeon who performed the operation (Haskins 1998). Usually flap observations should be performed at least every 15 min initially, then half hourly, hourly and finally 2–4 hourly. As the risk of venous and arterial thrombosis is greatest within the first 48–72 hours, postoperative monitoring is a crucial nursing function (Maksud 1992). The following information should be recorded, preferably using a flap observation chart. At shift changes the nurse should go through the flap observations with the nurse taking over this aspect of care to ensure that they are familiar with the flap's present condition.

Flap colour

This will depend on the colour of the skin at the site from which the flap was taken (Mahon 1987), e.g. in Caucasian's a free radial forearm flap used to reconstruct the tongue will be pale pink and therefore lighter in colour than the surrounding tissues. A fleshy pink is considered healthy in Caucasians but the darker the skin colour the more difficult it can be to assess (Coull & Wylie 1990, Coull 1992). A pale flap can indicate that the arterial supply is occluded, whereas a blue or purple coloured flap can indicate that the venous return is occluded (Edwards 1994, Adams & Lassen 1995).

Capillary refill

This is easily assessed by the application of gentle finger pressure to the flap to cause blanching of the skin, then releasing it and observing the time for capillary refill to occur (i.e. return to normal colour) (Coull & Wylie 1990). The tissue should blanch, then show return of colour within 3 s, timed from release of pressure (Mahon 1987). Slow or absent refill may indicate arterial problems (Coull & Wylie 1990, Coull 1992), whereas no blanching at all, or capillary refill of less than 1 s may indicate venous congestion (Edwards 1994). The plastic surgeon may request the use of a doppler (e.g. laser or ultrasound doppler) to monitor blood flow in the pedicle. The laser doppler sends a low power beam of laser light to the tissue through fibreoptics, providing a numerical or graphic display on the monitor of the average blood flow (Maksud 1992). The ultrasound doppler uses auscultation to identify a venous and an arterial tone (Westlake 1991). The surgeon will usually place a mark on the patient's skin over the pedicle artery during surgery to assist in the placement of the doppler probe. A 'whooshing' noise indicating blood flow can be heard when an ultrasound doppler is held over the artery.

Flap temperature

Ideally, the patient's temperature should be between 37 and 38°C, thereby ensuring that the flap is kept warm. As hypothermia can potentially cause vasoconstriction, which will impair the blood supply to the flap, room temperature should be maintained at or above 24°C (Westlake 1991, Edwards 1994). In order to assess flap temperature, Coull and Wylie (1990) suggest that, using one hand, one finger should be placed flat, palm upwards on the flap and another on the adjacent skin so a comparison can be made. A cool flap can indicate poor arterial flow, whilst an increasingly warmer flap can indicate reduced venous return or infection (Coull 1992). If gloves are required, the nurses caring for the patient should always use the same type of glove, as different thickness gloves may alter perception of the flap (Haskins 1998). Subdermal temperature electrodes may be preferred by some plastic surgeons. Electrodes are attached to the flap and to another area of tissue and a digital reading indicates the temperature. The flap temperature should be within 3°C of the comparative area of tissue (Westlake 1991).

Texture

The flap should be soft to touch. A distended, swollen or tense flap can indicate venous occlusion, whereas a hollow or dehydrated flap can indicate arterial occlusion (Maksud 1992, Edwards 1994, Adams & Lassen 1995).

Dermal bleeding (also known as pinprick response)

In addition to the above four flap observations, the plastic surgeon may request dermal bleeding to be assessed. This is performed by carefully inserting a sterile needle into the dermis of the flap. Moderate bleeding of bright red blood indicates that the flap is healthy (Westlake 1991). With venous congestion there is rapid bleeding of dark blood, while arterial occlusion will result in a minimal amount of dark blood or serum (Westlake 1991, Adams & Lassen 1995).

Flap dressings

Postoperative dressings must enable flap observations to take place. The dressing used must be sterile and absorbent, assist in containing exudate and enable the flap to be visualised clearly in order to detect changes in the flap's condition. For example, low-linting gauze with a window cut out and covered with an occlusive dressing, such as a semi-permeable film, will enable close monitoring of a flap.

Other points to consider

In addition to the specific flap observations described above, regular systemic observations and flap inspection must be performed. These additional points include:

(1) *Assessing fluid balance (including blood loss)* – Poor peripheral perfusion due to inadequate circulating blood volume will result in peripheral vasoconstriction and possible flap necrosis (Clamon & Netscher 1994).

(2) *Monitoring blood pressure* – Changes in blood pressure can affect the condition of the flap. For instance, hypotension may reduce arterial blood flow

resulting in a depletion of valuable nutrients, whereas hypertension may increase arterial flow resulting in congestion in the venous system of the flap (Coull & Wylie 1990).

(3) *Identifying infection* – Infection may produce flap necrosis. When combined with oedema, infection becomes an additional factor in causing the development of further necrosis (McGregor 1989).

(4) *Preventing kinking of the flap* – Kinking may create a blockage to the passage of blood across the line of the kink and can place strain on the pedicle of the flap, further compromising its circulation (McGregor 1989). Correct positioning of the patient is therefore essential to prevent kinking from occurring. By way of illustration, a patient with a flap repair to the head and neck should not be allowed to sleep with their head rolled towards the side of the flap (Haskins 1998).

(5) *Preventing tension* – Tension places the flap under considerable strain and causes hypo-perfusion of the flap (Haskins 1998).

(6) *Preventing pressure* – Pressure caused by bulky, tight dressings and tapes, e.g. tracheostomy tapes, can affect the viability of the flap and should therefore be avoided.

(7) *Maintaining the patency and vacuum of wound drains* – Patency should be checked regularly whilst performing other systemic and flap observations. Compression by a trapped haematoma on the vascular pedicle may result in flap necrosis (Clamon & Netscher 1994).

(8) *Educating the patient* – Educating the patient with regard to the implications of lifestyle behaviours on flap status is important, in particular tobacco smoking, which increases the possibility of platelet aggregation and hence the formation of blood clots (Coull & Wylie 1990). Decreased haemoglobin found in smokers means that inadequate blood oxygenation will slow down the healing process (Mahon 1987). Caffeine intake may also need to be reduced or discontinued if the flap blood supply appears compromised (Westlake 1991).

The early detection of any deterioration is essential as this enables prompt intervention to be carried out, such as the use of leeches, in order to save the flap. Care of surgical flaps therefore relies on a team approach between the plastic surgeons and nursing staff.

Leeches

Following the diagnosis of venous congestion in a flap, the plastic surgeons may prescribe the application of leeches. Without any intervention the arterial flow to the flap will diminish, eventually cutting off the blood supply and leading to tissue necrosis (Danton 1987). The leech species *Hirudo medicinalis* can produce a small bleeding wound which, due to special properties of the bite (which contains an anticoagulant, a local vasodilator and local anaesthetic), allows continued bleeding for up to 10 hours after the leech has detached (Biopharm 1996).

The patient, their family and some of the nursing staff may be unfamiliar with the use of leeches and will require support and information. The nurse will need to explain that the leeches are raised for this specific purpose and are never used on more than one patient (Peel 1993). Once the patient and family have learnt to appreciate the crucial role leeches will have in saving the flap, they may become more accustomed to this form of treatment. Some patients may prefer not to see the leeches *in situ*, whilst others may express more of an interest. Throughout the procedure it is essential for a nurse to remain with the patient, to provide reassurance and to monitor the leeches closely (Peel 1993).

Following the plastic surgeon's instructions on the frequency of application, the number of leeches to be used and the area on which to use the leeches, treatment can begin. Leeches are ordered from Biopharm UK, who provide detailed information on the maintenance, storage, use and disposal of leeches (Peel 1993). The area to be treated is cleaned with sterile water and then dried with sterile gauze (Voge & Lehnherr 1999). Skin preparations such as alcohol can prevent the leech from attaching and should therefore be avoided (Coull 1993, Voge & Lehnherr 1999). In accordance with local wound care policy and using an aseptic technique a leech is removed from the jar using long non-toothed forceps and placed on the area to be treated. The leech may need encouragement to latch on; this is done by making a small needle prick to produce a drop of blood, or by applying a sugary substance such as 5% glucose (Coull 1993). To prevent the leech from wandering the nurse should ensure that it attaches with both its anterior and posterior ends (Voge & Lehnherr 1999). Dressings or salt applied to non-treatment areas will also prevent the leech from wandering (Coull 1993). Leeches may remain attached for 30–60 min (Parker & Rendell 1994). Although the use of alcohol or saline will encourage the leech to detach, this could cause regurgitation leading to possible infection at the bite site (Adams & Lassen 1995). If the leech does not detach, once engorged it can be removed by paralysing it with topical cocaine (Wells *et al.* 1993). The used leeches are then disposed of by initially narcotising them with 8% alcohol, then placing them in 70% alcohol for 5 min before disposing of them via the sluice or an incinerator (Biopharm 1999).

Each bite wound will continue to ooze up to 150 ml of blood over the 10 h period after detachment (Biopharm 1999). Any blood clot formation should be removed to enable the wounds to continue to bleed freely (Coull 1993). The patient's haemoglobin should be monitored at regular intervals throughout the duration of treatment. Their temperature should also be monitored closely as the leech gut contains *Aeromonas hydrophilia* – a bacteria that is essential to the leech's growth and development. Although antibiotics can be prescribed, caution is advised, particularly when dealing with tissue that is, or is likely to become, compromised by poor arterial blood supply (Biopharm 1998).

SKIN GRAFTS

Definition

A skin graft is an area of skin that is completely separated from its site of origin, blood supply and nerve supply, and transplanted onto another anatomical site (Brown *et al.* 1998, Young & Fowler 1998).

Reference material

As a skin graft has no blood supply of its own, it is reliant on receiving oxygen and nutrients from the underlying blood vessels of its recipient site. A full thickness skin graft (FTSG), also known as a Wolfe graft includes the epidermis and all of the dermis, whereas a split skin graft (SSG) is composed of the epidermis and part of the dermis (Brown *et al.* 1998, Young & Fowler 1998). SSGs may be described as thin (Thiersch's graft), intermediate or thick according to the amount of dermis included and may be harvested from the patient (autograft), another human being (allograft) or another mammal, such as a pig (xenograft) (McGregor 1989, McCain & Sutherland 1998).

A skin graft may be used to repair extensive skin loss (e.g. from a burn), accelerate healing (e.g. chronic ulcer), reconstruct defects (e.g. a flap donor site) (Fig. 4.5) or close a surgical wound where direct closure with suturing is not possible (e.g. wide local excision) (Coull 1991, Young & Fowler 1998).

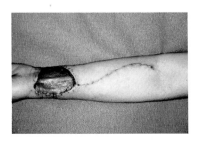

Fig. 4.5
Split skin graft on a free radial forearm
flap donor site.

Management of skin grafts

Split skin recipient site

A split skin recipient site is where the skin graft is applied. It may also be a flap donor site as a SSG is often used to cover areas from where a flap has been rotated or moved. The overall aim is to encourage the skin graft to attach and revascularise, collectively known as 'take' (McGregor 1989).

The patient usually returns from surgery with paraffin gauze or silicone net and surgical foam sutured or stapled in place over the graft (Balakrishnan 1994, Johnson *et al.* 1998). The former prevents dryness and adhesion whilst the latter provides thermal insulation thereby helping to maintain a warm, moist environment. This type of dressing also acts as a pressure dressing, provides protection and prevents shearing between the graft and its recipient wound bed (Balakrishnan 1994). The dressing is further secured with low-linting gauze and a crepe bandage or tapeless dressing and left undisturbed for 5 days. Movement of the graft site is restricted where appropriate to prevent any stress to the graft (Coull 1991).

Removal of postoperative dressing

On day 5, following the plastic surgeon's instructions, the outer dressing can be taken down and the sutures or staples securing the foam removed. Where appropriate the nurse should prepare the patient by describing the wound healing process, as the dressings will contain stale blood and exudate which can imply that the wound site will look the same. The foam and paraffin gauze silicone net is carefully lifted and separated from any SSG that may be adherent to it. If necessary sterile 0.9% sodium chloride can be used to facilitate the removal of the dressing. The SSG should be lying flat and be pink or red in colour. Any apparent seromas (collections of serous fluid under the SSG) should be expelled by using a sterile needle to evacuate the fluid. The graft is then carefully rolled from the centre outwards using sterile cotton buds to express any air, serous fluid or blood (Coull 1991). This action may be required twice daily in order to encourage the graft to take. Loose crusts or debris should be removed and any SSG that is overlapping the wound site trimmed back using fine forceps and scissors.

A paraffin gauze silicone net dressing is then reapplied to the graft, covered with low-linting gauze and a bandage. The pressure created from using this dressing can help express air or fluid from under the graft (Coull 1991). The dressing should be renewed daily or more frequently should visible 'strikethrough' occur (the presence of exudate on the outer dressing). The wound site should be observed daily for changes in exudate, colour and odour. Note that both *Streptococcus pyogenes* and *Pseudomonas aeruginosa*, which may be recognised by their distinctive bright green musty smelling exudate, may prevent graft 'take' if not treated promptly (Young & Fowler 1998). The SSG recipient site can be left exposed once exudate has diminished and seromas have disappeared. After healing, aqueous cream applied sparingly once or twice a day will keep the split skin supple.

Full thickness graft recipient site

FTSGs 'take' less easily in comparison to SSGs, as ideal conditions are necessary to support the graft, e.g. good vascularity and infection-free recipient site (Francis 1998). The graft site is generally secured using a 'tie over' dressing (a layer of foam sutured around the edge of the graft with the free ends of the sutures tied tightly across the top of the foam), which is removed as instructed by the plastic surgeon, usually after 5–10 days. An example of where a FTSG would be used is the excision of a basal cell carcinoma on the nose, which is repaired using a FTSG from the postauricular area.

Split skin donor site

This refers to the area from which the SSG is removed. The most common sites are the thighs, buttocks and upper arms (Fig. 4.6). The overall aim is to provide the optimum conditions to promote re-epithelialisation of the donor site (Rodzwic & Donnard 1986, Coull 1991, Wilkinson 1997). The donor site normally heals within 10–14 days (McGregor 1989). On return from surgery, the patient

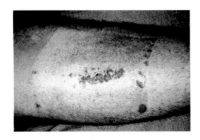

Fig. 4.6
Split skin graft donor site on the thigh.

will usually have an alginate dressing in place. This type of dressing is chosen for its haemostatic and absorbent properties (Thomas 1990) and is generally secured with low-linting gauze, cotton wool wadding and a crepe bandage or tapeless dressing. The combination of these dressings provides external pressure, which is initially required to assist with haemostasis (Wilkinson 1997). Regular analgesia should be given to the patient as the excision of the thin layer of skin leaves nerve endings exposed resulting in pain at the donor site.

Short term care of the donor site

(1) Low exudate
Where there is no evidence of 'strike-through' the dressing can be left alone. Occasionally, the dressing may slip exposing part of the wound site. In this instance the secondary dressing (bandage, cotton wool wadding and low-linting gauze) should be removed, enabling more alginate to be applied to the exposed site before reapplying a new, sterile secondary dressing. The bulk of the outer dressing can be reduced after 3–5 days if proving too cumbersome for the patient.

(2) Medium exudate
If strike-through is visible on the outer bandage the secondary dressings should be removed and replaced with new, sterile dressings while leaving the primary dressing in place.

(3) High exudate
This may indicate the presence of infection. Therefore the dressings should be removed and the colour and odour of the exudate observed, as donor sites can

also become infected by *Pseudomonas aeruginosa*. A wound swab should be taken to identify the infecting microorganism and its antibiotic sensitivities. The wound site should be cleaned with sterile 0.9% sodium chloride. Silver sulphadiazine 1% w/w (Flamazine®) cream should then be applied under a new sterile secondary dressing (Hamilton-Miller *et al.* 1993). Whilst infected the donor site should be checked daily and systemic antibiotics should be considered if the patient becomes unwell, e.g. raised temperature or increased donor site pain.

Long term care of the split skin donor site

On day ten following skin harvesting, the outer dressings should be removed and the primary alginate dressing assessed. If it is still firmly adherent to the donor site it should be left in place for a further 3–5 days and the outer dressings renewed. If however, the alginate dressing is loose in places and lifting off, it can be gently soaked off in a bath or shower, which will assist in minimising pain and trauma. Analgesia may be helpful if given to the patient prior to the dressing removal.

(1) Evidence of wound healing

A healing donor site is usually red, itchy and dry due to the loss of local sebaceous glands. Applying an aqueous cream twice daily will help to keep the area hydrated and supple. Any residual alginate fibres should be removed by using sterile 0.9% sodium chloride and forceps to prevent them becoming a focus for infection (Thomas 1990). The healing tissue will become paler and redness is usually minimal after 6 months (Wilkinson 1997). Where a further dressing is required, e.g. for patient comfort or to enable further wound healing, a hydrogel sheet may be used. These dressings feel cool and soothing, thereby helping to relieve pain and irritation (Thomas 1990). Where appropriate the dressing can be refrigerated (not frozen) to maximise the effect. The hydrogel dressing may be secured with gauze and a bandage and should be checked daily.

(2) Evidence of poor wound healing

A donor site that is red and raw with areas of bleeding indicates poor healing. An alginate dressing should be applied and covered with a secondary absorbent dressing such as low-linting gauze or pad and secured with a bandage. The wound site should be reassessed after 3–5 days.

Full thickness donor site

This refers to the area from which the FTSG is taken. Common sites include the postauricular, preauricular, supraclavicular, antecubital and inguinal areas, upper eyelid, scalp, hand, areola, prepuce and labia majora (Francis 1998). Closure of the FTSG donor site is usually achieved by direct closure with sutures; however, if this is not possible a SSG is applied to the donor site.

SCARRING

Definition

Scarring is the natural end result of tissue repair when damage extends beyond the dermis, and is defined as the misalignment of collagen fibres in the healed wound resulting in an altered appearance from normal skin (Eisenbeiss *et al.* 1998).

Reference material

One of the primary aims of wound care is to promote a healed wound that is cosmetically acceptable. When sutures or clips are still *in situ* the wound site must be observed regularly. By checking for the following signs and symptoms, prompt action can be taken which may prevent or relieve complications that, ultimately, could affect the cosmetic appearance of the scar line. The wound should be observed for:

(1) Signs of infection.
(2) Presence of purulent exudate.
(3) Signs of haematoma formation.
(4) Signs of actual or potential wound dehiscence.

Hypertrophic and keloid scars

Hypertrophic and keloid scars (Figs 4.7 and 4.8) are the result of an excessive fibrous tissue response (Williams 1996b). Keloid scars occur more frequently in darkly pigmented skin and are most likely to occur on the ear lobes, chin, neck, shoulders and upper trunk. Keloid scars consist of relatively large, parallel bands of densely collagenous material separated by bands of cellular tissue (Eisenbeiss *et al.* 1998). Characteristics of these scars are described in Table 4.1.

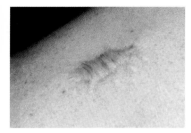

Fig. 4.7
A hypertrophic scar following excision of a mole.

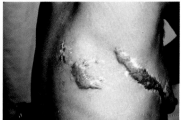

Fig. 4.8
Keloid scarring following Herpes zoster (shingles) of the T5/6 dermatomes.

Table 4.1 Characteristics of hypertrophic and keloid scars (Williams 1996b).

Hypertrophic scars (also known as protruding scars)	Keloid scars
(1) Usually occur soon after injury	(1) Usually occur some time after trauma or surgery
(2) Are more common in larger scars such as burns	(2) May develop from a small wound or minor surgery
(3) Have two growth phases, the first comprising active growth during which a smooth, solid scar forms, whilst the second phase consists of maturation and contraction	(3) Continue to grow for several years and spread, invading the surrounding tissue
(4) Are limited to the area of tissue damage	(4) Remain elevated and may be worsened by surgery

Management options

Finger massage

Finger massage can improve the condition of the scar and even assist in its disappearance. This should begin within days of the sutures being removed or when accompanying bruising has gone (Allsworth 1985). A bland cream such as E45 or a non-perfumed moisturising cream can be used to prevent friction between the finger and scar. The fingertips should be used in a tight circular motion working over the scar, paying attention to raised or hardened edges. It is important to use enough force to move the skin over the underlying structures. Ideally this should be performed for 10 min, six times each day (Allsworth 1985).

Pressure treatment

Pressure treatment is used for both keloid and hypertrophic scars. Elasticised garments are individually fitted and used to prevent contractures and to restore flatness and smoothness to scars, e.g. a Jobst garment that is worn following chest surgery. Pressure must be maintained for 12 months or longer, or until the scar has improved permanently (Davies 1985a, McGregor 1989). It is advisable that any breaks in pressure should not exceed 30 min per day (Munro 1995).

Intra-lesional steroid injection

Corticosteroid treatment appears to diminish tissue deposition and also to soften and flatten keloid scars (Munro 1995). Intra-lesional steroids reduce blood flow to the scar and promote the breakdown of collagen. It may be used on small scars but there is a risk of scar recurrence (Eisenbeiss *et al.* 1998).

Silicone gel sheet

Silicone gel sheeting can be used for the prevention and treatment of keloid and hypertrophic scars. The sheet softens, flattens and blanches scars (Williams 1996b). In a study on 42 patients with hypertrophic scarring silicone gel sheeting was found to be effective and safe (Carney *et al.* 1994). A silicone gel topical cream is also available (Silgel®) (Heenan 2000).

Glycerine-based hydrogel sheet

This dressing (Novogel® is the only one available at the time of writing) can be used for the prevention and treatment of hypertrophic and keloid scars. This sheeting has been shown to soften, flatten and relieve itching, redness and burning of scars (Baum & Busuito 1997). The product can be placed safely on open wounds at risk of abnormal scarring and is covered with a material backing which assists with conformity; however, it does require securing with tape, a secondary dressing or clothing (Baum & Busuito 1997).

Surgery

Surgical excision may be performed where a scar or lesion has grown taut resulting in a slight bulging effect in the surrounding tissue. A 'W' or 'Z' plasty may be performed where the scar is eased by cutting it in the line of relaxed skin tension (Allsworth 1985). For larger areas of scarring, surgical excision with or without skin grafting may be performed. Keloid scars, however, have a high rate of recurrence following surgery although the addition of postoperative radio-therapy may reduce the recurrence rate (Eisenbeiss *et al.* 1998).

Cosmetic camouflage

Cosmetic camouflage is most successfully used on those patients with atrophic (indented) and hypertrophic scars. Psychologically this service can benefit the client greatly (Allsworth 1985). Camouflage make-up is used to cover the scar so that it matches the surrounding skin tone. Advice and education are provided on the application and ordering of cosmetics, enabling the clients to develop their own skills. 'The role of the medical make-up specialist is to consult, observe, evaluate, design, educate and follow through' (Westmore 1991, p. 86).

GRAFT VERSUS HOST DISEASE OF THE SKIN

Definition

Graft versus host disease of the skin is an immune reaction initiated by the grafted bone marrow or stem cells against the host tissues of the graft reci-pient, with the skin as the target organ (McConn 1987, Buchsel 1997, DeMeyer *et al.* 1997).

Reference material

Acute graft versus host disease (GvHD) of the skin can appear within 10–70 days following bone marrow or stem cell transplantation. Chronic GvHD refers to reactions that occur over 3 months after transplantation (Aractingi & Chosidow 1998). The predominant causative agents for acute GvHD are the T-cells in the donated bone marrow, which react against the foreign antigens being expressed by the graft recipient's cells (Aractingi & Chosidow 1998). Eighty per cent of patients with chronic GvHD will have involvement of the skin (DeMeyer *et al.* 1997). GvHD of the skin may present in a number of forms including an erythematous rash, blistering, cracking and/or weeping of the skin (McConn 1987, Buchsel 1997).

The primary aim of managing GvHD of the skin is to maintain the integrity of the skin as far as possible in order to minimise the risk of infection. This is best achieved by cleansing and moisturising the skin. The use of daily warm baths with bath oil and a cream based soap (as opposed to a deodorant soap) is recommended (McConn 1987).

The breakdown of skin integrity and associated altered body image can have a substantial psychological impact on the patient and their family or caregiver. It is imperative that continuing support, care, information and co-operation is provided to avoid psychological morbidity. Involvement of the multidisciplinary team is vital to ensure the best care for the patient (DeMeyer *et al.* 1997).

Management options

The following management options are recommended for broken skin or skin at risk of breaking down.

Blistering

(1) Intact fluid-filled blisters
- Leave alone.
Or, if painful
- Apply a hydrogel sheet.

(2) Burst and open blisters
Treat as an open wound and apply:
- Hydrogel.
- Hydrogel sheet.
- Alginate dressings.

(Do not apply a hydrocolloid sheet as the surrounding, friable skin may also breakdown when the dressing is removed).

- If a burning sensation is present apply silver sulphadiazine cream (Flamazine®) and cover with a secondary low-adherent dressing.

Cracked dry or bleeding skin
The skin may be cracked and dry or bleeding due to 'shedding' of keratinised epithelial cells.

- Moisturise with oilatum washes and apply an emollient cream or petroleum jelly.

And/or, if painful

- Apply a hydrogel sheet.

Cracked, weeping skin
- Apply a foam sheet dressing.

For extensive areas of skin breakdown a specialised burns foam or dressing may be applied to provide a non-adherent and protective layer to minimise the risk of infection (e.g. Exu Dry® – Smith & Nephew™).

ACUTE SKIN REACTIONS TO RADIOTHERAPY

Definition
Acute skin reactions to radiotherapy are characterised by local irritation, erythema, dry flaky skin, or moist sloughing of the epidermal layers over the area of skin within the radiotherapy treatment field (Thomas 1992a, Bennett & Moody 1995). See also Table 4.2.

Table 4.2 Categories of acute radiotherapy skin reactions.

Category	Description
Erythema	Reddened skin, which may be oedematous and feel hot and irritable
Dry desquamation	Reddened skin that is dry, flaky or peeling and may be itchy
Moist desquamation	Peeling skin with exposure of the dermis accompanied by exudate production. Often painful and may become infected
Necrosis	Skin may darken and turn black and/or form a non-healing ulcer

(Campbell & Lane 1996, Boot-Vickers & Eaton 1999)

Reference material

The effect of ionising radiation on living cells is to cause damage to their intracellular components resulting in a disruption of cell division and cell death. The DNA is very sensitive to damage by radiation, particularly when it is exposed during cell division. The maximum effect of radiotherapy therefore occurs just before and during cell division, hence cell populations with a high rate of division are prone to radiation damage (Copp 1991, Hilderley 1997). Cells that have undergone malignant changes divide at an abnormally increased rate thus making them highly susceptible to the effects of radiation (Tortora & Grabowski 1996, Weinberg 1996). However, many normal cell populations have a naturally high cell division rate and the effect of radiation upon these cells causes many of the side effects associated with radiotherapy treatment. These cells are found in a number of body sites including the mucous membranes (mouth, intestines and vagina), bone marrow and skin (Souhami & Tobias 1998).

During radiotherapy treatment of superficial or deep tumours the skin always receives part of the radiation dose. Irradiation of the skin damages the rapidly dividing cells in the basal layer of the epidermis (stratum basale) preventing the normal process of replacing the outer, keratinised, cells (Hopewell 1990, Bennett & Moody 1995, Campbell & Lane 1996). There is usually an initial inflammatory reaction, evidenced by erythema of the skin, which may be followed by dry or moist desquamation (Table 4.2) (Hopewell 1990, Thomas 1992a, Bennett & Moody 1995, Campbell & Lane 1996). Skin reactions tend to occur more frequently in areas of friction or increased moisture such as the axilla, inframammary fold and perineum (Rigter *et al.* 1994, Blackmar 1997). Although it is very uncommon with modern radiotherapy treatment methods, the most severe reaction that may occur is the development of ischaemia, due to capillary damage, and subsequent skin necrosis (Hopewell 1990). It should be remembered that the skin will not heal until the radiotherapy treatment has finished (Campbell & Lane 1996).

There is little systematic research investigating the efficacy of different regimes of radiotherapy skin care (Thomas 1992a, Barkham 1993, Lavery 1995). The guidelines presented here are therefore based on logical principles derived from the best evidence available. This includes study results, published opinions from leaders in the field and expert views of professionals within The Royal Marsden Hospital.

Aims of acute skin reaction management:

(1) To preserve skin integrity.
(2) To provide psychosocial and educational support to the patient.
(3) To provide comfort to the skin.
(4) To minimise symptoms arising from radiotherapy skin reactions.
(5) To provide optimum conditions for healing.

Skin reactions to radiotherapy may be severe and patients will often require psychosocial support and education throughout and after treatment to assist them in minimising, and coping with, the associated symptoms. In addition, patients should be reassessed regularly and actual or potential radiotherapy-related symptoms managed appropriately.

Management options
Management includes preventative measures as well as treating actual skin reactions.

Assessment
A thorough assessment is required prior to the patient starting radiotherapy and should include the following:

(1) The presence of high risk factors for acute radiation induced skin reaction
- High total dose of radiation.
- Low energy radiation or electrons.
- Treatment of the head and neck, breast or pelvic area.
- Large volume of normal tissue included in the area of treatment.
- Tangential treatment fields.
- Use of 'bolus' materials (e.g. a wax blanket to increase the dose of radiotherapy to the skin).
- Older age.
- Immunosuppression.
- Concurrent chemotherapy or steroid therapy.
- Poor nutritional status.
- Tobacco smoking.
- Chronic sun exposure.

(Goodman *et al.* 1997, Porock *et al.* 1998)

(2) Baseline skin assessment
- Current skin condition.
- Concurrent skin disorders.
- Surgical changes (e.g. scars).

(3) Educational needs of the patient and their family or carers
- Information on treatment details and potential side effects.

(Copp 1991, Goodman *et al.* 1997)

Preventative measures

To help avoid adverse skin reactions patients should be advised to take preventative measures during radiotherapy treatment (Campbell & Illingworth 1992). It may be helpful to provide the patient with an information sheet on care of the skin during radiotherapy (Fig. 4.9).

Management options

Management depends on the presenting skin reaction features and is described below according to the different skin reaction categories.

Erythema and dry desquamation

Erythema may occur within 2–3 weeks of commencing radiotherapy (Fig. 4.10) (Copp 1991, Goodman *et al.* 1997). Treatment of dry desquamation is the same as for erythema. The aims of management are to prevent skin breakdown and relieve symptoms of burning and itching. This may be achieved by:

(1) Preventing further skin irritation by following the advice outlined in Fig. 4.9.
(2) Moisturising the skin with an emollient cream.

If pruritis and/or pain are present:

(3) Applying topical steroid cream (1% hydrocortisone) for irritation or itching (should be applied sparingly).
(4) Applying cooled hydrogel sheets.

(Boot-Vickers & Eaton 1999)

Moist desquamation

The care of moist desquamative skin reactions (Fig. 4.11) is based on the principles of moist wound healing. Management should encompass the following points:

Skin care information sheet for patients having radiotherapy treatment

You may develop a skin reaction during your radiotherapy treatment. It will look similar to sunburn and may be red, sore and itchy. Your Doctor, Nurse or Radiographer will be able to help if the skin is dry, painful or weepy. The skin reaction may last for 2 to 4 weeks after your treatment has finished. By following the suggestions below you should be able to reduce the possibility of developing or worsening a skin reaction. You should continue to follow these suggestions until your skin is completely healed.

Your Doctor, Nurse or Radiographer will be happy to answer any questions or concerns you have about your treatment.

- Wash normally using warm water. You may use a non-perfumed, mild soap on the treated skin.
- Pat your skin dry with a soft towel.
- Ensure any treatment field marks (ink pen marks) are not removed.
- Apply a moisturising cream to the skin two to three times a day to help maintain its softness. Your Doctor, Nurse or Radiographer can suggest a good moisturiser (..).
- Avoid the use of deodorants and perfumed skin care products in the treated area.
- Avoid the use of flannels, brushes, loofah etc. on the treated area, as these may damage the skin.
- Wear loose comfortable clothing. Underwear should be the correct size and natural fibres such as cotton are recommended.
- Protect the treated skin from extreme cold and sunlight during treatment. Once treatment has finished continue to protect the skin from sunlight until any skin reactions have subsided. Once the skin has fully healed you should continue to protect it from strong sunlight. A high protection factor sunscreen (15+ or greater) is recommended, or cover the skin with clothing to protect it.
- Continue your usual activities during treatment whenever possible. However some activities, such as swimming, should be discussed with your Doctor or Nurse if your skin reaction becomes worse.
- Eat a balanced diet and drink plenty of fluids throughout treatment. If eating or drinking is difficult talk to your Doctor or Nurse who will be able to help.
- Further specific advice _____
  _____
  _____

Fig. 4.9 Patient information sheet on skin care during radiotherapy.

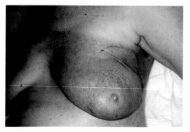

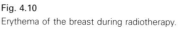

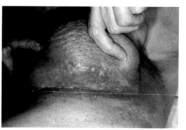

Fig. 4.10
Erythema of the breast during radiotherapy.

Fig. 4.11
Moist desquamation in the inframammary fold of the breast during radiotherapy.

(1) Wound assessment

- Assess and record wound dimensions, colour, appearance and the nature of any exudate.
- If signs of infection are evident (e.g. underlying cellulitis, delayed healing, severe discomfort and/or increased exudate) a microbiology swab of the wound should be taken and the patient referred to medical staff as systemic antibiotic therapy may be required.

(2) Wound management

- Commence with thorough irrigation of the wound (either with sterile 0.9% sodium chloride or by showering).
- The choice of dressing is dictated by the amount of exudate produced by the wound and also by the fact that the dressing must be removed prior to treatment (see Tables 4.3 & 4.4).

Note: Minimise the use of adherent materials within the treatment field. Products that are suitable for securing dressings include lightweight elastic conforming bandage (e.g. Netelast® or Tubifast®) or the use of underwear, such as sports or maternity sleeping bras, or crop tops.

Table 4.3 Wound dressings for moist desquamation.

Treatment phase	None or low exudate production	Moderate to high exudate production
During treatment	• Hydrogel sheets • Hydrogel or hydrocolloid gel	• Foam sheets • Hydrofibre sheets • Alginate sheets (useful if bleeding is present)
	(note: these dressings must be removed each treatment)	
Post-treatment	• Hydrogel sheets • Hydrocolloid gel or hydrogel • Hydrocolloid sheets	• Foam sheets • Alginate sheet (plus secondary dressing) • Hydrofibre sheet (plus secondary dressing)

ADDITIONAL ADVICE FOR SPECIFIC SKIN AREAS

Breast

(1) During treatment

Skin reactions tend to occur after about 3–4 weeks of treatment. The following factors can exacerbate skin reactions:

• Previous surgery – the scar line may be more prone to problems.
• Previous and concurrent chemotherapy.
• Large and/or pendulous breasts are prone to reactions in the skin folds.
• Wearing ill-fitting bras, particularly wired or elasticised bras.
• Use of a wax sheet.

The radiographer will advise whether or not dressings can be left in place during treatment. Generally dressings should be removed before treatment to prevent a build-up of radiation dose to the skin. However, exceptions to this may be made for some patients with fungating chest wall lesions, where it may be advantageous to increase the dose of radiotherapy to the skin. The extra layer of the dressing will increase the dose to that area. However, the same type of dressing will need to be used throughout treatment and will need to be in place during the treatment planning phases.

Table 4.4 Quick reference guide to acute radiotherapy skin reaction management.

| | During radiotherapy treatment | | | | |
| | No exudate | | Exudate | | |
Type of skin reaction	No discomfort	Discomfort	Low	High	Infection* additional measures
Erythema	Emollient cream** Baby formulation talcum powder	Emollient cream** Baby formulation talcum powder Hydrocortisone 1% cream			
Dry desquamation	Emollient cream**	Emollient cream** Hydrogel sheet*			
Moist desquamation			Hydrogel sheets* or hydrogel + Secondary dressing	Foam sheets or hydrofibre or alginate (if bleeding) + Secondary dressing	Microbiology swab Oral antibiotics as indicated Daily dressing changes required
Necrosis	Refer to necrotic wound section Chapter 3				

* Geliperm® (hydrogel sheet) should not be used with a *Pseudomonas* infection
** Examples: Aqueous cream, E45®

Post-radiotherapy treatment				
No exudate		Exudate		
No discomfort	Discomfort	Low	High	Infection* additional measures
Emollient cream** Baby formulation talcum powder	Emollient cream** Hydrocortisone 1% cream			
	Hydrogel sheets			
Emollient cream**	Emollient cream** Hydrogel sheets Hydrocolloid sheets			
		Hydrogel sheets* or hydrogel or hydrocolloid sheets	Alginate or hydrofibre +/– foam sheet +/– secondary dressing	Microbiology swab Oral antibiotics as indicated Daily dressing changes required

(2) Post-treatment
Maximal reactions tend to occur 7–10 days after completion of treatment. If the skin has broken down, it generally heals rapidly once treatment has finished. Where appropriate patients should be advised to wear a well-fitting bra (sports bras or maternity sleep bras are often useful). However, comfort is a priority and some patients may prefer not to wear a bra at all.

(3) Securing dressings
It is often difficult to secure dressings in these patients, particularly in large and/or pendulous breasted patients where the skin folds are affected. Tapes should be avoided as the adhesives can damage fragile skin. Therefore soft bras, crop-tops and vests made from lightweight elastic conforming bandage (e.g. Netelast®) are recommended as an alternative means of securing dressings.

Pelvis

Pelvic radiotherapy will often include the genitals and rectum within the treatment field.

(1) During treatment
Patients should be assessed on an individual basis and their treatment and care planned accordingly. Patients treated with parallel opposed fields, i.e. beams from front and back, are at an increased risk of skin reactions compared to those receiving treatment with multiple fields, i.e. three or more, as the dose per field is less in the latter. Skin reactions usually occur after about 4 weeks of treatment.

Areas at an increased risk for acute skin reactions, due to increased moisture and friction, include:

- Natal cleft.
- Groins.
- Skin folds.
- Perineum.

Problems other than skin reactions may occur and need specific care. These include:

(a) Vaginal discharge
Patients are offered regular douching with warm tap water, both during and after treatment. This promotes comfort, reduces odour and decreases discharge.

(b) Vaginal bleeding

Douching should be stopped until bleeding is under control and the cause is found.

(c) Vaginal stenosis

Radiotherapy changes the lining of the vagina. It may become fibrosed and less elastic. Vaginal lubrication and dilators are required to maintain patient comfort (Rice 1997).

(d) Severe skin reactions and local oedema

Patients having radiotherapy to the vulva often require a break from treatment because of severe skin reactions and local oedema.

Note: Patients receiving concurrent chemotherapy and radiotherapy are susceptible to more severe vaginal or scrotal skin reactions.

Head and neck

During planning, patients have individual moulds and plastic shells prepared to immobilise their head during treatment. This extra layer can increase the dose of radiotherapy to the skin surface. Parts of the shell may be removed to reduce this effect (skin sparing). This is particularly important if the patient has any scars or biopsy sites, which are more prone to a reaction, as these will almost always be inside the treatment field and, therefore, under the shell.

(1) During treatment

Wet shaving, perfumed skin products and fitted collars should all be avoided to minimise local skin irritation. Skin folds are particularly vulnerable to skin reactions (e.g. behind the ears).

(a) Hair loss

Men should be advised to shave beards and moustaches before mould or shell fitting. All patients should be made aware that any hair within the treatment field might be lost permanently. Patients may wash their hair with a mild, non-medicated shampoo throughout treatment. In order to prevent tugging of the hair roots and surrounding skin, patients should be advised to use a soft bristle hairbrush, avoid vigorous rubbing and not to use hair rollers. In addition, to minimise any further risk of damage to the scalp by the application of heat, the use of hairdryers, heated rollers etc. should be avoided.

(b) Mucositis
Radiotherapy to the head and neck often causes severe mucositis (inflammation of the oral mucosa) and therefore exacerbates the problems of maintaining an adequate nutritional intake. This is a particular problem for patients with pre-existing eating difficulties. Poor nutritional status can lead to an increase in skin reactions and delayed healing. An appropriate referral to a dietician, prior to the patient starting treatment, is essential.

(2) Dressing choice
It should be remembered that these patients may already have facial disfigurement and therefore a sensitive approach to dressing choice is essential.

(a) Securing dressings
It is often difficult to secure dressings to the head, face and neck area. The emphasis should be on comfort and minimising bulky dressings. The use of natural fibres, such as silk scarves, is often a useful way of securing dressings.

(b) Post-treatment
Hydrocolloid sheets are often a good choice as they are thin, do not require secondary dressings or tapes to secure, blend in better with most skin tones and can be left in place for long periods.

FUNGATING WOUNDS

Definition
A fungating wound develops from the extension of a malignant tumour into the structures of the skin producing a raised or ulcerating necrotic lesion (Fig. 4.12) (Moody & Grocott 1993, Bennett & Moody 1995). They are generally characterised by the 'lip' that surrounds the margin of the wound and by the very nature of their complexity.

Reference material
'Each malignant ulcer is unique, requiring individual assessment. Treatment should be realistic and accepted by the patient and carers. If the treatment

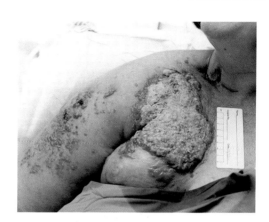

Fig. 4.12
A large fungating breast
wound with multiple
nodules present on the
upper arm.

does not promote quality of life and a sense of well being, it should be changed. Few treatments are absolute. When the prognosis is short (days) the primary aim should be to promote comfort.'

(Saunders & Regnard 1989, p. 153)

Aetiology and incidence

Tumour infiltration of the skin may develop either from direct invasion by a local tumour or through metastatic spread into the epithelium, capillaries or lymph vessels of the skin. As the tumour enlarges it causes the capillaries to rupture or become occluded, resulting in necrosis of the skin and subsequent formation of a cutaneous wound (Moody & Grocott 1993, Bennett & Moody 1995). These wounds often become infected, produce offensive smelling exudate and bleed very easily (Hampton 1996). Common tumours associated with fungating wounds are breast carcinoma, sarcoma, squamous cell carcinoma and melanoma (Fig. 4.13) (Hallett 1995b). Radiotherapy, chemotherapy and hormone therapy may have some effect on reducing the size and symptoms of these wounds but the benefits of these treatments need to be balanced against their potential side effects.

Fungating wounds present many challenges to nursing staff because they rarely heal and they produce a multitude of problems which are often recurring and difficult to manage (Laverty *et al.* 2000a). Management is based on symptom control and maintaining or improving quality of life (Laverty *et al.*

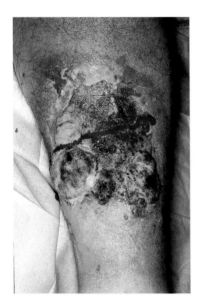

Fig. 4.13
Fungating lesions on the lower posterior
leg from malignant melanoma.

1997, Laverty *et al.* 2000a). This is best achieved through the use of a holistic
assessment, psychosocial support and appropriate use of dressing products
(Saunders & Regnard 1989, Moody & Grocott 1993, Bennett & Moody 1995,
Haisfield-Wolfe & Rund 1997).

There has been little research into the incidence of fungating wounds. The
most commonly quoted study was conducted by Thomas (1992a) who sent
questionnaires to all of the radiotherapy centres in the UK. He reported that, for
all of these centres, there were around 295 patients with fungating wounds
seen in 1 month and approximately 2417 patients were seen in 1 year. He con-
cluded, 'fungating wounds occur in sufficient numbers to represent a significant
problem' (Thomas 1992a, p. 6). Approximately 5–10% of cancer patients with
metastatic disease will develop a fungating lesion, with around 62% arising from
breast cancer (Thomas 1992a, Haisfield-Wolfe & Baxendale-Cox 1999). Patients
aged from 60 to 70 years old are most affected and the wounds usually
occur in the last 6 months of life (Ivetić & Lyne 1990, Haisfield-Wolfe & Rund
1997).

Aims of management

The plan of care should include an overall aim. In the case of fungating wounds, where healing is unlikely, the focus of care should be:

(1) Comfort.
(2) Improve quality of life.
(3) Control symptoms.
(4) Promote confidence and a sense of well being.

(Lister 1991, Moody & Grocott 1993, Haisfield-Wolfe & Rund 1997)

This should involve planning to use dressings and/or interventions that promote these aspects of care. It may be useful to discuss the patient's previous experiences with dressing products and non-pharmacological interventions in order to gain insight into their effectiveness.

Management options

These wounds have a number of problems, which can be ameliorated by the type of dressings used. It is imperative that the patient is assessed holistically in order to address all issues relating to the wound.

Physical symptoms

Fungating wounds usually present with multiple symptoms (Laverty 2000a). Often, when one problem is resolved, a new one is likely to take its place.

The main presenting physical symptoms include:

(1) Slough/Necrosis.
(2) Infection.
(3) Exudate*.
(4) Malodour*.
(5) Bleeding*.
(6) Pain (at wound site).
(7) Itching/irritation.

* Denotes those symptoms identified by patients as being the most distressing

(Collinson 1992)

While addressed individually here, it is important to remember that these symptoms often occur together, and therefore cannot be managed in isolation (Laverty *et al.* 2000a). Generally, fungating lesions do not heal; therefore it may be unnecessary to use dressings that promote optimum conditions for wound healing. However, the maintenance of a moist wound environment should be encouraged if possible. The priorities for dressing choice should be:

(1) Patient comfort and acceptability.
(2) Minimising slough and necrotic tissue.
(3) Minimising infection.
(4) Containing odour.
(5) Containing exudate.

Slough/necrosis

The purpose of removing slough and/or necrotic tissue is to lessen the risk of infection occurring. There are a number of different types of debridement that may be used; however, some of them are not appropriate for these patients due to their invasive nature (e.g. surgical or sharp debridement).

(1) Enzymatic debridement

This may be considered but it is costly and extreme caution is required due to the likelihood that the enzyme preparation will be taken up systemically; therefore its use is not recommended on actively bleeding wounds, which is often the case with fungating lesions.

(2) Debridement by autolysis

This is a much more acceptable and less invasive treatment. The principle is to provide a moist environment by using a product that can donate fluid and absorb excess fluid in a gentle manner by promoting autolysis (destruction of tissue) of slough/necrotic tissue (Bale 1997).

(3) Larval therapy

Recently more interest has been reported in support of this treatment. The larvae (fly maggots) are placed in the wound bed where they act by rapidly cleansing the wound of necrotic and sloughy material (Thomas *et al.* 1998a). A case study has explored the use of larval therapy in a sloughy, malodorous malignant wound with good effect (Jones *et al.* 1998a). The thought of having the maggots placed in the wound may be offensive for the patient and their use is generally reserved for more acute wounds.

Note: Refer to the sections on necrotic and sloughy wounds in Chapter 3 for more information on the use of the different debridement techniques.

Infection

Due to the chronic nature of fungating wounds, a sudden increase in the patient's wound symptoms may be the first indicator of wound infection (Gilchrist 1999). Generally, a wound swab will confirm the presence or absence of infection in the wound (see section on infected wounds in Chapter 3). Systemic antibiotics may be used in treating the infection; however, blood supply to fungating wounds is often poor and the concentration of antibiotic at the wound site may not be sufficient to have any effect.

Exudate

Exudate is probably the most common problem associated with fungating wounds. Wound exudate contains nutrients and energy for metabolising cells and, most importantly, maintains a moist environment, which promotes healing. However, too much exudate can cause maceration of skin and may be very distressing due to the difficulties with containing the fluids and preventing leakage from the dressings. Fluid production becomes more viscous and malodorous in infected wounds and prompt treatment is required. A great deal of clinical experience in this area has highlighted the fact that profuse exudate can cause enormous embarrassment to the patient due to the risk of leakage. Staining of clothes and bed linen are frequent problems and need to be addressed sensitively. In addition, patients may express feelings of being unclean and dirty and have a reluctance to share a bed with their partner. The nurse can play a valuable role in addressing these issues by selecting the most effective dressing and actively listening to the concerns, worries and priorities of the patient and their family or caregiver.

Dressings used to contain exudate should have minimal bulk, whilst preventing leakage and creating an acceptable cosmetic effect (Thomas 1997). Dressings have different absorbency properties and it is important to select the correct dressing, although this will need to be reviewed at each dressing change (Thomas 1997). Protection of the surrounding skin is also of vital importance to prevent breakdown and enlargement of the wound. Suitable products for exudate control are presented in Table 4.5.

Table 4.5 Suggested products for the management of exudate in fungating wounds.

Low exudate wounds	High exudate wounds	Protection of surrounding skin
• Hydrocolloid sheets • Semi-permeable films • Low adherent, absorbent dressings	• Alginates/hydrofibre • Foam dressings • Low adherent wound contact layer plus secondary absorbent pad • Stoma appliances	• Hydrocolloid sheets (picture framing wound) • Skin barrier films and creams • Adequate dressing overlap

(Cooper 1993, Grocott 1998, Jones *et al.* 1998)

Malodour

The presence of this pervasive odour can lead to embarrassment, disgust, depression and social isolation (Van Toller 1994, Finlay *et al.* 1996, Jones *et al.* 1998b). Malodour is usually due to the breakdown of proteins in dead tissue by anaerobic bacteria, therefore debridement is important (Bale 1997). The main aims of management are to kill the anaerobic organisms that are responsible for the odour formation and to filter out any malodour.

(1) Metronidazole

Metronidazole kills the bacteria responsible for odour production (Ashford *et al.* 1980, Newman *et al.* 1989, Bower *et al.* 1992). Systemic treatment may be helpful, but side effects such as nausea, alcohol intolerance and neuropathy have been reported with oral therapy (Hampton 1996). Sparrow *et al.* (1980) found that a dose of 200 mg orally three times a day was as effective in controlling malodour as 400 mg orally three times a day but with fewer side effects. When systemic treatment is not possible, topical metronidazole gel (0.75% or 0.8% w/v) can be used (Cutting 1998, Gilchrist 1999). A treatment course of 5–7 days should be sufficient to control the odour. However, the problem frequently recurs and further courses will probably be necessary (Thomas 1992a, Hampton 1996).

Metronidazole gel can be mixed with a hydrogel, in equal quantities, to combine the properties of odour and slough management (SMTL 1999).

(2) Activated charcoal dressings
These can be used in conjunction with metronidazole gel. They are usually used as a secondary dressing as contact with moisture renders them ineffective (Bennett & Moody 1995, Haisfield-Wolfe & Rund 1997, SMTL 1999). However, there are now several dressings available that contain a layer of activated charcoal as well as an absorbent primary wound contract layer (e.g. CarboFlex®, Lyofoam C®).

(3) Sugar paste and honey
These products produce a hyperosmotic environment that inhibits bacterial growth. Honey contains other antibacterial components as well. They may also promote debridement of the wound (Morgan 1997, Cooper & Molan 1999).

(4) Natural live yoghurt
There is little research to support the use of live yoghurt but it may help to debride the wound and prevent the growth of bacteria, thereby encouraging healing. It also lowers the pH of the wound environment (Schulte 1993). The yoghurt is applied to the wound and left for 10 minutes then thoroughly rinsed off before applying an appropriate dressing.

(5) Occlusive dressings
These dressings can be used to contain exudate and prevent the escape of wound malodour (Thomas 1998).

(6) Daily dressing changes/disposal of soiled dressings
This practice prevents the build-up of stale exudate.

(7) Deodorisers
Includes essential oils, environmental air filters and commercial deodorisers. These may be more useful once the odour is controlled, but may not be effective in masking an odour. Commercial deodorisers may make the odour worse or cause unpleasant associations with smells.

Bleeding

Bleeding in fungating wounds can be related to tumour activity or due to the application of inappropriate dressings. Care must be taken to ensure that if a dressing is adherent to the wound it is irrigated well to avoid any trauma. Bleeding may also be affected by decreased platelet function within the tumour. It is important to observe the amount of blood loss so that adequate measures, such as a blood transfusion (if appropriate), can be taken in the event of a large bleed (Dealey 1999).

The psychological distress caused by a heavy bleed can be devastating for the patient, family and the health care professionals involved. If there is a risk of a bleed, consideration needs to be given as to where the patient would be cared for best. It may be inappropriate for care to continue at home especially if there are young children in the house and/or if the patient, carer or family do not feel they can cope.

(1) Light bleeding or oozing of blood
- Alginate dressings can be applied directly to bleeding areas of an otherwise dry, open wound provided the dressing is first moistened with a little sterile 0.9% sodium chloride solution. This will prevent the alginate drying out and adhering to the wound causing pain and further bleeding on removal (Thomas 1990, Bennett & Moody 1995).

(2) Profuse bleeding
Immediate measures should be taken such as:

- Application of a haemostatic surgical sponge (e.g. Spongostan®).
- Adrenaline solution (1 in 1000 for injection) applied topically (can cause ischaemic necrosis due to vasoconstriction).
- Oral or topical application of tranexamic acid solution (for injection).
- Cauterisation of bleeding vessels; this measure is rarely performed now due to the availability of effective dressing products.
- Ligation of bleeding vessels by a surgeon.
- Application of silver nitrate, although this can cause blackened skin and irregularities in the urea and electrolyte levels in the blood, therefore it is rarely used.
- Application of sucralfate cream.
     (Jash 1973, Haisfield-Wolfe & Rund 1997, Emflorgo 1998, Dealey 1999, Bird 2000, Laverty *et al.* 2000a)

Radiotherapy may also be used as it destroys the tumour cells, which leads to a reduction in tumour mass and a consequent reduction in symptoms (Capra 1986, Young 1997). This is usually given as a single dose.

Pain

Pain is generally a protective function (Casey 1998). In fungating wounds, pain is often due to the erosion and breakdown of the nerve endings, which cannot be repaired. Pain may be acute due to further invasion/growth of the tumour or chronic due to the damage already sustained. If pain occurs during dressing changes it may be due to adherence of the dressing. Thorough irrigation to soak the dressing may ease removal, and a review of the choice of dressing may be necessary (Lister 1991, Moody & Grocott 1993). The assessment of pain from the wound site should be managed separately from any other pain that the patient is experiencing. For chronic pain, appropriate analgesics should be chosen in accordance with prescribing policies and guidelines.

(1) Local anaesthetic agents
Local anaesthetic agents act by blocking the action potential (the message of pain that reaches the brain), for example lignocaine gel, which can be applied directly to the wound surface (Rang 1995).

(2) Opioids
The use of a short acting strong analgesic during dressing changes ensures that pain relief is effective but short-lived and therefore has fewer side effects (e.g. dextromoramide) (Pilsworth *et al.* 1995). On the other hand a breakthrough dose of the patient's usual analgesia (e.g. oral morphine sulphate or hydromorphone hydrochloride) can be used but it has longer lasting effects post dressing.

(3) Topical opioids
Diamorphine or morphine can be mixed with a carrier gel, such as a water-soluble medical lubricant (e.g. KY Jelly®) or a hydrogel, and applied directly to the wound surface. It has been suggested that the process of inflammation causes peripheral nerve endings to produce opioid receptors and will also produce endogenous opioid peptides, thus making the wound sensitive to topical opioids (Stein 1995). Discussion also surrounds the question of whether

morphine and diamorphine have an anti-inflammatory effect or a true analgesic effect. It is not clear whether the intensity of the inflammation is relevant to the degree of opioid action (Back & Finlay 1995, Stein 1995).

(4) Entonox administration
There is no research evidence to support its use in wound management but because it is a short acting method of managing pain, and because expert opinion and clinical experience supports it use, it is frequently utilised (Peate & Lancaster 2000).

(5) Non-steroidal anti-inflammatory drugs (NSAIDs)
Non-steroidal anti-inflammatory drugs can be useful if pain is associated with local inflammation (e.g. diclofenac sodium and ibuprofen). Caution should be exercised due to NSAIDs severe gastro-intestinal side effect profile (Rang 1995).

(6) Local skin barrier
Pain may be due to skin maceration and excoriation by exudate, hence a protective skin barrier will reduce pain (MacGregor *et al.* 1994, Hampton 1998). Examples include Cavilon®, Superskin® and Lutrol.

Itching

This is often a chronic problem when tumour nodules are beginning to emerge under the surrounding skin. The stretching of the skin irritates nerve endings and may cause a biochemical reaction leading to local inflammation.

(1) Hydrogel sheets
These have a cooling effect when applied to itching irritable skin, which can be enhanced if the dressing is stored in a non-food refrigerator. Apply the gel sheet to the wound surface and cover with a secondary dressing, such as a semi-permeable film, to prevent dehydration of the dressing, or, if the wound is producing exudate, cover with a dry dressing and secure in place.

(2) Menthol in aqueous cream
This is an alternative to calamine lotion but does not dry out on the skin. Menthol has a cooling effect. Menthol in aqueous cream can be applied to itching areas two or three times a day or more frequently if necessary. It should not be applied to areas of skin loss where nodules have broken down.

Which management option?

Dressing choice should be based primarily on the appearance of the wound bed and should follow the previously described management of necrotic, sloughy, granulating or infected wounds and include the management strategies outlined above for specific symptoms (Figs 4.14a to 4.14f). The choice of dressing should be regularly reviewed according to the patient's condition and any discussion on management options should involve the patient and their carers (Bennett & Moody 1995, Mallett & Dougherty 2000).

SUPPLY AND ADMINISTRATION OF WOUND MANAGEMENT PRODUCTS

At present only certain nurses holding district nurse or health visitor qualifications who have completed an approved prescribing course are allowed to pre-

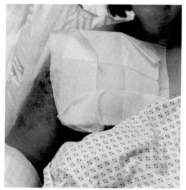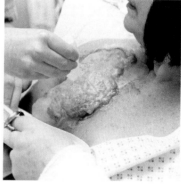

(b)

Fig. 4.14 (a–f) While fungating wounds can be complex and difficult to manage, a well thought out management strategy can make wound care simpler. This series of photographs demonstrates the process of changing a dressing on a sloughy, malodorous fungating breast wound. The initial dressing (a) is composed of an alginate that is covered by a hydrocellular foam sheet and secured with fabric retention tape; note that the tape has lifted and there has been leakage at the bottom of the dressing. The wound is irrigated with warmed 0.9% sodium chloride (b) to remove the alginate and cleanse the wound. Metronidazole gel is applied to the wound to control malodour (c) and a new dressing of a self-adhesive hydropolymer foam is applied (d and e). The final dressing is thinner and more comfortable than the original but still highly absorbent and the self-adhesive border will reduce the risk of any leaks (f). Consent for publication kindly given by the patient.

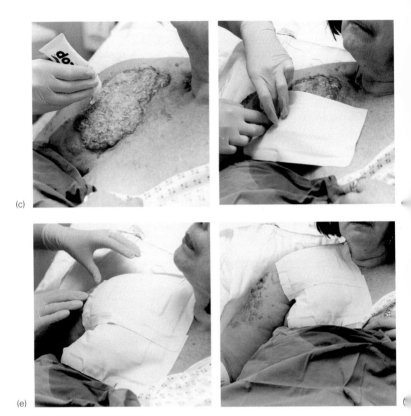

(c)

(e)

Fig. 4.14 (a–f) *Continued*

scribe from a limited formulary (DoH 1999, see also Dougherty *et al.* 2000). This situation is likely to change in the future (see DoH 1999); however, until this time many nurses (and other professionals) are utilising Patient Group Directions to supply and administer medicines in order to support their practice.

Patient Group Directions (PGD), also known as Group Protocols, are specific written instructions for the supply and administration, or administration, of a named medicine in an identified clinical situation. Directions apply to groups of patients who may not be individually identified before presenting for treatment. The Direction should be drawn up locally by doctors, pharmacists and relevant health professionals as appropriate and approved by the employer advised by the relevant professional committees (DoH 1998, MCA 2000).

Patient Group Directions have been used at The Royal Marsden Hospital for a number of years to underpin nursing initiatives, such as nurse-led clinics (Laverty *et al.* 1997, Mallett *et al.* 1997). They have recently been developed further to encompass the recommendations in the Crown Report relating to Group Protocols – *Review of Prescribing, Supply and Administration of Medicines. A Report on the Supply and Administration of Medicines under Group Protocols* (DoH 1998). The resultant document was a generic 'framework' for patient-focused Group Protocols that could be utilised for the supply and administration of medicines, including some prescription-only medicines (PoMs) (Dougherty *et al.* 2000).

In order to facilitate wound management, a PGD has been developed for the management of fungating wounds via the supply and administration of wound management products (see Appendix). This provides a guide for nurses according to the patients' symptoms and the condition of the wound, as well as allowing for the appropriate administration of items such as hydrocolloids, alginates, debriding enzymes and metronidazole gel (the latter two being PoMs). The PGD also includes sections on the audit trail, competency of the nurse and authorisation of the Directions. At the time of press this PGD is about to go into use and be evaluated via the audit trail. It is anticipated that the PGD will assist nurses in ensuring best practice in wound management for patients with cancer.

PSYCHOLOGICAL, SEXUAL AND SOCIAL PROBLEMS RELATED TO CHRONIC WOUNDS

The focus on the physical symptoms in wound care should not undervalue the importance of the many psychological aspects that arise when a chronic wound is present. As previously stated, the assessment of the wound should include not only physical but the psychological, spiritual, cultural and social aspects as well. Good communication is vitally important and the ability to listen effectively is essential so that these issues can be fully and sensitively explored. Counselling skills and coping mechanisms should be fully utilised when helping patients and their families come to terms with the presence of a chronic and/or complex wound.

The distress caused by a chronic wound will vary depending on the individual and the impact the wound has upon their quality of life and ability to function normally (Figs 4.15a, 4.15b and 4.15c). For example, if a patient has to give up

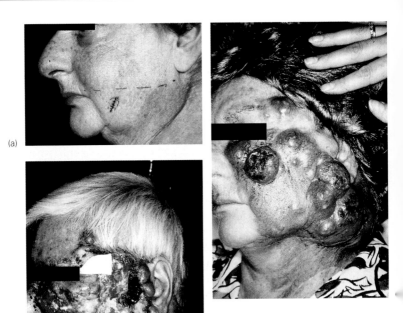

(a)

(c)

Fig. 4.15 (a–c) Fungating wounds can have a devastating effect on the social and psychological well being of patients, particularly when the wound occurs on a highly visible part of the body. This 62 year old woman (Mrs J.) presented with a small nodule on her check which was excised (a) and found to be a Merkel cell tumour. Mrs J. was a very outgoing lady who was married with two children and four grandchildren. She lived an active lifestyle and took pride in her appearance. Two years later the tumour had progressed and was beginning to fungate and break down (b). Mrs J's husband was finding it hard to cope with her changed appearance and her grandchildren were frightened of her; she was becoming very reclusive and isolated. Three months later Mrs J. was admitted to the palliative care unit following a large spontaneous bleed from the wound, which had deteriorated considerably (c), and she died a few weeks later.

their work or restrict their social life because of symptoms related to their wound, it may have an enormous influence on their outlook (Collinson 1992). There are many obstacles created due to the presence of a wound and one of the main concerns tends to be the physical management of the wound and the implications for the patient and family (Collinson 1992). This may mean that the patient has to wait in the home for the arrival of community staff who dress the wound, disrupting any social arrangements that the patient would like to make and also making it impossible for the person to go to work.

Relationships can be severely affected (Bird 2000). The sharing of common facilities may cause immense embarrassment and symptoms such as odour and excessive exudate may lead to reluctance to go to bed with their partner due to the likelihood of leakage and staining of the patient's clothes or bedding during the night (Grocott 1995, Laverty *et al.* 2000a). Patients may find the continuation of the physical side of a relationship extremely difficult. Hallett (1995b) and Haughton & Young (1995) suggest that the social stigma, guilt and shame associated with a malodorous wound can have a negative influence on a patient's emotional state and may have a detrimental effect on sexual expression leading to relationship problems. These issues need to be handled in a very sensitive and appropriate manner. Addressing the physical problems may help the patient deal with the psychological consequences by a process of adaptation and can be of extreme value. For example, considering innovative ways of securing dressings may be beneficial in boosting the patient's self-esteem, and the effective management of wound exudate leads to increased levels of patient confidence and comfort (Haisfield-Wolfe & Rund 1997).

As in most cases of chronic disease, the level of useful practical interventions may be limited, but the patient's lifestyle and personal issues will require constant attention and review. Additional interventions enabling the patient to cope, such as the use of complementary therapies (e.g. relaxation, distraction techniques, aromatherapy, etc.) can be useful (Bird 2000).

No two patients will cope with a wound in the same way, and an individual assessment without any underlying presumptions or prejudice is the mainstay of an ideal management strategy. In considering the situation these patients face Doyle (1980, in Ivetić & Lyne 1990, p. 87) aptly wrote: 'Can we begin to imagine what it must feel like for a patient to see part of his body rotting and to have to live with the offensive smell from it, see the reactions of his visitors (including doctors and nurses) and know that it signifies lingering death?'

Outcomes/evaluation

Normally the evaluation of a wound would be dependent upon the degree of healing. With fungating and other chronic wounds the goal is different and therefore the outcomes should be measured against the aims of care as discussed previously in this chapter. The patient should be the key person in evaluating the care given, as they are the most appropriate judge of the effectiveness of care. Evaluation should be from both physical and psychosocial standpoints. The physical aspect includes whether or not wound care products have been effective in managing and controlling symptoms. From a psychosocial perspective, have the physical management, communication skills and the general advice given by the health care professional enabled the patient, and their family or carer, to live as full a life as possible? The original outcome targets should have been set by all those involved in the patient's care, especially the patient themselves. It is these targets that further assessments should be measured against, with the targets being reviewed and altered as necessary.

The final part of evaluation leads back to assessment. Is it possible to improve on the original goal and aim for a further achievable target? Frequently this may not be possible because of the recurrence or worsening of previous symptoms or an unresolved initial issue. Management of chronic wounds, in particular fungating wounds, often involves compromise due to the very nature of the patient's deteriorating health. The health care professional will need to exercise tact and patience in working with the patient and their family or carer to set realistic goals and, if necessary, to deal with the consequences of not achieving them.

CONCLUSION

Chronic and complex wounds create an enormous challenge for all health care professionals who are involved in the patient's ongoing management. It is clear that there is not one dressing that is the ultimate answer to the patient's needs (Grocott 2000), nor is the practical management of the wound the complete picture. Attention needs to be given to ongoing, continuous assessment that involves the patient's understanding and overall coping abilities. The communication demonstrated by the health care professional plays a large part in gaining and retaining the patient's trust and building a relationship that can be nurtured.

5

A Guide to Wound Management Products

Introduction

The products available for wound care have changed and developed considerably since the first experiments with occlusive film dressings in the 1960s (Gelbart 1999). There is now a large and diverse array of products available made from materials that range from seaweed to silicone. With the multitude of products and treatments available and new ones constantly being developed, choosing the right dressing can be a confusing experience for many health professionals. As an aid to dressing and treatment choice this chapter explores these different products, what they are and when to use them. The products are grouped under their generic names, such as hydrocolloids or alginates, but it should be remembered that the various products in each category will have different performance characteristics. The products covered include the more fundamental dressings and treatments that have definite applications in oncology patients and not those that may still be considered 'experimental', such as growth factors or skin substitutes.

Note: in this chapter an asterisk (*) indicates dressing products used within The Royal Marsden NHS Trust at the time of writing.

ACTIVATED CHARCOAL DRESSINGS

Description

Activated charcoal dressings contain a layer of activated charcoal (Fig. 5.1) that traps volatile, odour-causing molecules from the air, thereby reducing or removing the smell of malodorous wounds (Thomas *et al.* 1998b).

Reference material

While most activated charcoal dressings simply absorb odour, some also kill bacteria (e.g. Actisorb Silver 220®). However, it should be noted that they are not a replacement for active treatment of the underlying cause of the odour, which is usually due to a bacterial infection (Thomas *et al.* 1998b). These

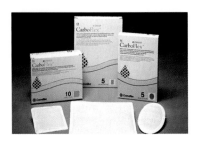

Fig. 5.1
An activated charcoal dressing with alginate/hydrofibre wound contact layer (photograph kindly supplied by ConvaTec Ltd). Reproduced from material provided by ConvaTec Ltd.

dressings are available as secondary dressings or as primary wound dressings, some of which contain other dressing materials, for example alginate and hydrofibre mix (e.g. CarboFlex®).

Examples
Clinisorb®*, Denidor® (secondary dressings), Actisorb Silver 220®, CarboFlex®, Kaltocarb®, Lyofoam C® (primary wound dressings).

Indications
- Malodorous wounds, including fungating tumours, faecal fistulae, necrotic pressure ulcers and leg ulcers (SMTL 1999).

Contra-indications
- Depends on dressing constituents; secondary dressings have no contraindications.

ADHESIVE ISLAND DRESSINGS

Description
Adhesive island dressings consist of a low adherent, absorbent pad located centrally on an adhesive backing (Fig. 5.2). The backing may consist of a non-woven polyester fabric, a semi-permeable film or permeable polyurethane (Morgan 1997).

Reference material
Adhesive island dressings are generally used for postoperative management of suture lines although they may also be used for low exudate superficial wounds.

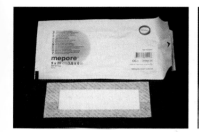

Fig. 5.2
An adhesive island dressing. Reproduced from material provided by Mölnlyche Healthcare Limited.

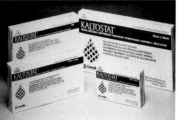

Fig. 5.3
An alginate dressing (photograph kindly supplied by ConvaTec Ltd). Reproduced from material provided by ConvaTec Ltd.

Examples

Mepore®*, Opsite Post-Op®, Primapore®, Tielle Lite®.

Indications

• Lightly exuding wounds.
• Postoperative wounds.

Contra-indications

• Known sensitivity to dressings or their adhesives.
• Fragile or easily damaged skin.
• Heavily exuding wounds.

(Thomas Hess 1998, SMTL 1999)

Precautions

• Do not apply the dressing under tension as the shearing forces produced may damage the skin.

ALGINATES

Description

Alginates are a textile fibre dressing made from the calcium salt of an alginic acid polymer derived from brown seaweed (Fig. 5.3). They contain mannuronic and guluronic acids in varying amounts and are available as a sheet, ribbon or packing (Thomas 2000).

Reference material

Calcium alginate, in contact with serum, wound exudate or sodium-containing solutions, is converted to soluble sodium alginate and forms a hydrophilic gel which overlays the wound and provides an environment that promotes healing (Thomas 1990, Williams 1994, Heenan 1998). Alginates that have high levels of mannuronic acid (e.g. Sorbsan®) form soft flexible gels on contact with wound exudate, while those high in guluronic acid (e.g. Kaltostat®) are more cohesive and form a more solid gel (Morgan 1997). Alginates that form soft gels are more easily irrigated out of wounds, while those that remain more cohesive can be removed from a wound in one piece.

Some patients experience a mild tingling sensation when the dressing is first applied due to 'drawing up' of surface exudate. Moistening the wound surface with a little sterile 0.9% sodium chloride solution can prevent this side effect (Thomas 1994, SMTL 1999). Removal of alginates may be facilitated by irrigation with 0.9% sodium chloride solution to increase gel formation thereby reducing adhesion that may cause trauma to the wound bed and discomfort to the patient (Thomas 1990).

Examples

Comfeel Seasorb®, Curasorb®, Kaltostat®, Sorbsan®*, Tegagen®.

Indications

- Moderate to highly exuding wounds (sloughy, granulating).
- Infected/malodorous wounds.
- Bleeding wounds, including skin donor sites; alginates have haemostatic properties (although not all alginates have a product licence for this use).
- Painful wounds where other dressings have adhered to tissue.

(Thomas 1992b, SMTL 1995, Heenan 1998, SMTL 1999)

Contra-indications

- Dry wounds.
- Dry necrotic areas (eschar).

(SMTL 1999)

DEBRIDING ENZYMES

Description
Debriding enzymes usually consist of a mixture of the two enzymes, streptokinase and streptodornase (Rutter *et al.* 2000).

Reference material
Streptokinase liquefies blood clots, fibrin and fibrinogen, and streptodornase liquefies nucleoproteins from dead cells or pus (Hampton 1999a, Rutter *et al.* 2000). The most commonly used enzyme preparation in the UK is Varidase®(Fig. 5.4), which is presented as a vial of sterile powder that must be stored in a refrigerator (Morgan 1997).

Example
Varidase®*.

Indications
- Removal of hard necrotic material resistant to hydrogel.
- Removal of dry or adherent slough resistant to hydrogel.
- Infected wounds.

(Morgan 1997)

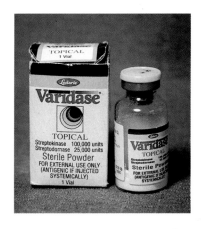

Fig. 5.4
An enzyme preparation (Varidase®).
Reproduced from material provided by
Wyeth Laboratories.

Contra-indications

- It should not be used on actively bleeding wounds.
- Patients with hypersensitivity to streptokinase or streptodornase.
- Patients who may be at risk of coronary artery disease.

(Poston 1996)

FOAMS

Description

Foam dressings are available in a variety of forms (Fig. 5.5). They are generally made from polyurethane foam and may have one or more layers. A silicone polymer foam cavity dressing is also available. Foam dressings are absorbent, non-adherent and provide a moist, thermally insulated wound environment (Bale & Harding 1991, Young 1998).

Reference material

The different types of foam dressings are described here under the separate headings of silicone polymer foam, polyurethane foam and hydrosorbtive dressings.

Silicone polymer foam

Silicone polymer foam consists of two liquid components, a polymer suspension and catalyst. When combined they release hydrogen causing the mixture to expand and form a soft, pliable, non-adherent, absorbent, white foam (Thomas 1990).

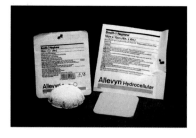

Fig. 5.5
Hydrocellular foam sheet and cavity dressings. Reproduced from material provided by Smith & Nephew Healthcare Limited.

Example
Cavi-Care®*.

Indications
- Granulating cavity wounds.
- Sloughy cavity wounds (used in combination with a hydrogel).
- Surgically produced cavities, for example pilonidal sinus drainage, open perianal or perineal wounds.

    (Thomas 1990, Bale & Harding 1991, Williams 1995b, SMTL 1999)

Contra-indications
- Deep narrow wounds that may contain hidden sinuses or pockets. There is a danger that small pieces of foam may become detached and remain undetected in the wound.
- Mucous membranes, for example eyes and nose.

    (Williams 1995b, SMTL 1999)

Precautions
- The wound must be open with no hidden pockets and the opening larger than the base.
- Any current treatment for necrotic/sloughy or infected tissue must continue, as the dressing itself will not remove these symptoms.
- During preparation, wear gloves and avoid contact with eyes and clothing.

    (SMTL 1999)

Polyurethane foams
These foams generally consist of soft, highly absorbent polyurethane foam and may be presented with or without an adhesive surface or border. There are several types of foam dressing available in two main categories, hydrocellular and hydropolymer.

Hydrocellular foams
Hydrocellular foams come in a number of forms; firstly, as a three-layered dressing consisting of a perforated, non-adherent polyurethane film 'wound contact' layer, a middle layer of highly absorbent polyurethane foam and an outer layer of semi-permeable polyurethane film (e.g. Allevyn®, Spyrosorb®). The outer film

prevents strike-through of exudate and the passage of microorganisms (Thomas 1990). Hydrocellular foams are also available as cavity dressings consisting of polyurethane foam chips encapsulated in a honeycombed polyurethane film, and available in circular and tubular shapes with two sizes of each shape (e.g. Allevyn Cavity®) (Bale & Harding 1991, Williams 1995a, SMTL 1999).

Hydrocellular foams are available in another form as an open cell, hydrophobic, polyurethane foam sheet that has had one side heat-treated to collapse the foam cells and form a wound contact layer that absorbs exudate through capillary action (e.g. Lyofoam®) (Williams 1999b). Excess fluid then evaporates from the open cell side of the dressing. This type of hydrocellular foam dressing is available as variously sized sheets and also as a tracheostomy and drain site dressing (e.g. Lyofoam T®*) with a pre-cut 'keyhole'.

Examples

Allevyn®*, Allevyn Cavity®*, Lyofoam®*, Spyrosorb®.

Hydropolymer foam

Hydropolymer foams are available as island dressings consisting of a polyurethane backing which is permeable but waterproof, a non-woven wicking layer and a highly absorbent polyurethane foam wound contact layer (e.g. Tielle®). The hydropolymer foam swells as it absorbs fluid, with excess fluid being absorbed into the wicking layer and vented by the permeable backing. These dressings are also available with a superabsorbent viscose/rayon and acrylate wicking layer, which forms a gel on contact with fluid and is able to absorb and contain large amounts of wound exudate (e.g. Tielle Plus®) (Hampton 1999a, Johnson & Johnson Medical 2000).

Examples

Tielle®, Tielle Plus®*.

Indications

- Light to moderately exuding superficial wounds.
- Cavity wounds (Allevyn cavity®).
- Tracheostomy and drain sites (Lyofoam T®, Allevyn Tracheostomy®).
- Hypergranulation (Lyofoam®).
- May be used under compression dressings.

(Bale & Harding 1991, SMTL 1999)

Contra-indications
- Dry necrotic wounds.
- Wounds with low exudate.
- Shallow, drying wounds (due to possible adherence).
- Heavily exuding wounds (except Tielle Plus®).

(SMTL 1999)

Precautions
- Infected wounds.
- Allevyn Cavity® should not be re-used.
- Allevyn Cavity® should not be cut open.
- Do not soak Allevyn Cavity® dressings in oxidising agents such as Eusol or hydrogen peroxide as these break down the foam filling.

Hydrosorbtive dressings
Hydrosorbtive dressings are a recent development and are slightly different from the normal foam dressings. The wound contact layer is non-adherent, the central core is composed of super-absorbent granules in powder form and the backing layer is a thin hydrocolloid sheet (Morgan 1997, Thomas 1997). Exudate is absorbed and locked into the dressings central core.

Examples
CombiDerm®*, CombiDerm N®*.

Indications
- Chronic or acute moderately exuding wounds.
- Clean granulating wounds.
- Necrotic or sloughy wounds.
- Infected wounds (not an ideal choice as it needs to be changed daily, making treatment expensive).

(SMTL 1999)

Contra-indications
- Known sensitivity to hydrocolloid or its components.

HONEY

Definition

Honey is produced by bees from flower nectar, which may be collected from a variety of flowering plants and trees. As a wound care product it is available as impregnated dressing pads and tubes of liquid honey and has many beneficial properties that make it useful as a wound dressing (Molan 1999a).

Reference material

Honey is one of the oldest recorded dressings used by man, being used in wound care over 4000 years ago (Molan 1999b). It has an antibacterial action that is attributed to several sources. Firstly, the highly osmotic nature of honey absorbs water in the wound leaving none free for bacterial growth (WHRU 1996). Secondly, the presence of hydrogen peroxide, which is slowly released by the honey as it becomes diluted in the wound, is highly bacteriocidal (Molan 1999a). Several honeys have also been found to contain plant-derived antibacterial agents (Morgan 1997). In addition, honey provides a moist wound environment and is non-adherent causing no trauma to the wound on removal (Molan 1999b). It also promotes debridement of the wound and helps to eliminate wound malodour. This latter action may be due to bacteria using sugars in the honey in preference to proteins from necrotic tissue (Molan 1999d). Honey has an anti-inflammatory effect that is unrelated to its antibacterial action and may be attributed to the presence of antioxidants in the honey (Molan 1999b).

Honey aids wound healing in other ways; for example the presence of hydrogen peroxide in the honey is thought to stimulate the formation of granulation tissue and re-epithelialisation of the wound. Honey also produces an acidic environment that promotes wound healing, and it contains amino acids, vitamins, trace elements and sugars which provide a ready source of nutrients to the healing tissues (Molan 1999d).

The antibacterial effect of honey is most helpful on infected wounds and it has been shown to be effective against antibiotic resistant bacteria including MRSA (Molan 1999d). This is becoming increasingly important as more bacteria develop antibiotic resistance. The antibacterial and debriding effects of honey are ideal for the palliative treatment of fungating wounds where it reduces inflammation and exudate production and has a rapid deodorising effect.

Honey is available in different consistencies, but stirring or warming will alter its thickness, although it should not be heated over 37°C as this will affect the antibacterial function of the honey and may burn the patient (Molan 1999d). Honey used in wound care should be sterilised by gamma irradiation, as there is the possibility of clostridium spores being present in the honey that could cause wound botulism (Postmes *et al.* 1993, Molan 1999d). It is preferable to use a honey specifically manufactured for use in wounds.

The amount of honey used on a wound will depend on the level of exudate and infection present. High levels of exudate will dilute the honey and reduce its effectiveness. Severe infection will need more honey in order to have an effect. Usually 30 ml of honey is used per 10 cm^2 of dressing pad (Molan 1999a). Honey has no harmful effects on healing tissues and no allergic reactions have been reported, only very rare cases of stinging or pain on application (Molan 1999c).

Indications
- Infected wounds (including abscesses).
- Necrotic and sloughy wounds (including gangrenous wounds).
- Chronic wounds.
- Burns.
- Fungating wounds.
- Surgical wounds, in particular infected surgical wounds and vulvectomy wounds.
- Pre-skin grafting.

(Subrahmanyam 1991, Morgan 1997, Molan 1999b, Molan 1999d)

Contra-indications
- Diabetes is the only contraindication for the use of honey due to the absorption of glucose and fructose (Morgan 1997). However this is debatable, as it has been used successfully in the treatment of diabetic foot ulcers (Molan 1999b).

HYDROCOLLOIDS

Description
A hydrocolloid consists of a wound contact layer (base material) containing amounts of gelatin, pectin and carboxymethylcellulose combined with

adhesives and polymers. The hydrocolloid base material may be bonded to either a semi-permeable film, or a semi-permeable film plus polyurethane foam, and may or may not have an extra, adhesive border (Fig. 5.6) (Bennett & Moody 1995, Jones & Milton 2000b).

Reference material

In the presence of wound exudate the hydrocolloid base material forms a semi-solid gel (Jones & Milton 2000b). Hydrocolloid dressings are self-adhesive and waterproof and therefore should not require a secondary dressing. In areas where movement could loosen the edges of the dressing, for example on the sacrum, a bordered hydrocolloid may be more appropriate. Alternatively an adhesive retention dressing may be useful (e.g. a semi-permeable film or retention sheet) although this may alter the moisture vapour transfer rate of the hydro-colloid causing maceration of the surrounding skin (Jones & Milton 2000b). Different hydrocolloid dressings have particular properties and should be chosen for their suitability to the wound they will be used on.

Examples

Comfeel®, Duoderm E®*, Granuflex®*, Hydrocoll®, Tegasorb®.

Indications

- Light to moderately exuding wounds.
- Clean granulating wounds.

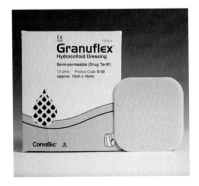

Fig. 5.6
A hydrocolloid dressing (photograph kindly supplied by ConvaTec Ltd). Reproduced from material provided by ConvaTec Ltd.

- Necrotic or sloughy wounds.
- Infected wounds (not an ideal choice as it needs to be changed daily, making treatment expensive).

(SMTL 1999)

Contra-indications

- Known sensitivity to hydrocolloid or its components.
- Highly exuding wounds. Hydrocolloids are not recommended for use in these wounds as the frequency of dressing change makes a hydrocolloid sheet uneconomical.

(Thomas 1990, SMTL 1999)

HYDROGELS

Description

Hydrogel dressings contain from 17.5 to 90% water plus various other components depending on the type and manufacturer (see below). They are capable of absorbing excess exudate while also donating fluid to dry necrotic areas (Jones & Milton 2000c).

Reference material

These dressings are available in two forms, firstly as amorphous gels that slowly lose their cohesiveness as they absorb fluid, and secondly as flat sheets that maintain a three-dimensional structure (Fig. 5.7) (Bennett & Moody 1995, Miller & Dyson 1996).

Amorphous gels

Amorphous hydrogels contain differing quantities of water and propylene glycol plus other components, such as sodium carboxymethylcellulose or alginate, depending on the product. Hydrogels that contain high levels of pectin and sodium carboxymethylcellulose have the properties of both hydrocolloids and hydrogels. They are able to hydrate tissue while maintaining an absorptive capacity as well as having good cohesive properties (Williams 1996a, SMTL 1999). Hydrogels require a secondary dressing.

Examples

Aquaform®, Granugel®*, Intrasite Gel®, Nu-Gel®, Purilon®, Sterigel®.

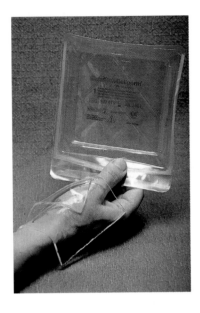

Fig. 5.7
A hydrogel sheet dressing. Reproduced from material provided by Geistlich Pharma.

Indications

- Deep or superficial wounds.
- Rehydration of eschar.
- Sloughy wounds with light to moderate exudate.
- Granulating wounds (to maintain a moist environment to encourage granulation and epithelialisation).
- Protection and comfort of fungating lesions.

(Williams 1996a, SMTL 1999, Jones & Milton 2000c)

Contra-indications

- Known sensitivity to the gel or its components.
- Heavily exuding wounds.

(Williams 1996a, SMTL 1999)

Precautions

- Infected wounds (hydrogels can be used alongside systemic antibiotic treatment with close monitoring for any deterioration of the wound).

- Occlusion is not recommended in the presence of anaerobic infection.
- Safety is not yet established in third degree burns.

(Williams 1996a, SMTL 1999)

Hydrogel sheets

Hydrogel sheets generally contain between 60 and 96% water or isotonic saline, the remainder being composed of varying amounts of different agents depending on the product. These may include polyethylene oxide, agar, polyacrylamide, polyurethane polymer and propylene glycol. They are permeable to oxygen, water vapour and small protein molecules, but impermeable to bacteria. They provide a moist, well-oxygenated environment and have cooling properties (Thomas 1990, Morgan 1997, SMTL 1999). Hydrogel sheets feel cold and moist to touch and are very soothing when placed on irritated skin; refrigeration of the dressing will enhance this effect (Morgan 1997). One hydrogel sheet dressing is glycerine based rather than water based (Novogel®). It is composed of 65% glycerine, 17.5% polyacrylamide and 17.5% water with an outer layer of stretch Lycra. It is absorbent (three to four times its own weight in fluid) and is also bacteriostatic and fungistatic. Novogel® will not dehydrate, as most other hydrogel sheets do, and forms a comfortable match against body contours (Southwest Technologies Inc 2000).

Examples

Geliperm®*, Novogel®*, Clearsite®, Hydrosorb®, Spenco 2nd Skin®, Vigilon®.

Indications

- Shallow, clean wounds with limited damage.
- Light to moderately exuding wounds.
- Acute radiotherapy skin reactions.
- Superficial nodules of fungating lesions causing irritation.
- Split skin donor sites.
- Recipient graft sites.
- Superficial pressure ulcers.
- Deep chronic wounds extending to muscle, tendon or bone.
- Fungating and/or malodorous wounds (Novogel®)..

(Thomas 1990, SMTL 1999)

Contra-indications

- Wounds known to be infected (particularly with *Pseudomonas aeruginosa*).
- Deep narrow cavities or sinus wounds.
- Patients with known hypersensitivity to glycerine (Novogel® only).

(Thomas 1990, SMTL 1999)

HYDROFIBRE

Description

A hydrofibre is a soft, non-woven dressing composed of 100% hydrocolloid fibres (sodium carboxymethylcellulose) (Williams 1999a).

Reference material

Hydrofibre dressings are available as a sheet or ribbon (Fig. 5.8) and are highly absorbent; hydrofibre is able to take up to 30 times its own weight in fluid. It provides a moist wound healing environment while keeping excess wound drainage locked within its structure, preventing maceration of surrounding skin (Williams 1999a, Robinson 2000). Hydrofibres form a cohesive, clear gel on contact with wound fluids.

Example

Aquacel®*.

Indications

- Moderate to highly exuding acute and chronic wounds.
- Cavity wounds.
- Wounds prone to bleeding.

(Hallett & Hampton 1999, SMTL 1999, Williams 1999a)

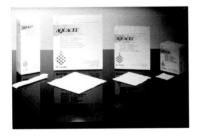

Fig. 5.8
A hydrofibre dressing (photograph kindly supplied by ConvaTec Ltd). Reproduced from material provided by ConvaTec Ltd.

Contra-indications

- Known sensitivity to hydrofibre or its components.
- Dry, necrotic wounds.

(SMTL 1999, Williams 1999a)

LARVAL THERAPY

Description

Larval therapy is the application of fly larvae (maggots) to a wound to remove necrotic sloughy tissue and treat infection (Fig. 5.9) (Sherman 1996).

Reference material

Larval therapy (also referred to as biosurgery) is not a new concept; it was first described in 1579 and again during the 1800s and was also used in both World War I and II (Sherman 1996, Thomas *et al.* 1999b). In early accounts, larval infestation was usually by accident. But in the early 1900s to the 1940s maggots were intentionally introduced into wounds with various dressings and devices used to keep the maggots in the wound; they were also bred for use in hospitals in America (Thomas *et al.* 1998a). The introduction of antibiotics saw a decline in the use of larval therapy until recently with the emergence of antibiotic-resistant bacterial strains (Thomas *et al.* 1999a).

The Biosurgical Research Unit at Bridgend Hospital in Wales currently produces sterile larvae on a commercial basis. The species they breed is *Lucilia sericata* or the common greenbottle blowfly (Biosurgical Research Unit 1999). This species was chosen for a number of reasons. Its lifecycle has been well

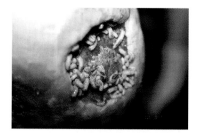

Fig. 5.9
Larval therapy being used to debride a pressure ulcer on the heel of a diabetic patient (photograph kindly supplied by Dr S. Thomas).

documented and the larvae produce powerful enzymes that break down dead tissue, but they do not invade healthy tissue (Thomas *et al.* 1998a). The larvae debride slough and necrotic tissue and at the same time they remove bacteria from the wound (Thomas *et al.* 1999b). Their use has led to reduced odour and pain from wounds and the promotion of wound healing (Sherman 1998).

As long as the patient agrees to the therapy, the use of maggots is considered an ethical treatment. However, while it may be unacceptable to both patients and staff, the usefulness of larval therapy in wound management should not be overlooked.

Sterile larvae (marketed as Larv E) can be ordered from the Biosurgical Research Unit and are delivered by courier along with a container of sterile saline and nylon net retention dressing. The larvae should be used within 8h of delivery and should be stored in a cool dark place until required (Biosurgical Research Unit 1999).

Indications

Larval therapy may be used on almost any type of sloughy, necrotic or infected wound:

- Malignant fungating wounds.
- Abscesses.
- Infected surgical wounds.
- Leg ulcers.
- Diabetic ulcers.
- Pressure ulcers.
- Burns.
- Osteomyelitis.
- Necrotising faciitis.

(Gacheru 1998, Jones *et al.* 1998a, Thomas & Jones 1999)

Contra-indications

- Wounds that may bleed easily or where there are exposed large blood vessels, because of the risk of erosion by larval enzymes.
- Fistulae or wounds that connect with body cavities or organs.

(Thomas & Jones 1999)

METRONIDAZOLE GEL

Description

Metronidazole gel is a clear, colourless, sterile gel containing 0.75 or 0.8% w/v metronidazole in an aqueous base (Fig. 5.10) (Morgan 1997).

Reference material

Metronidazole is active against anaerobic bacteria that are associated with odour production in fungating or chronic wounds. At the concentrations achieved topically it is also active against some organisms which would otherwise be resistant to metronidazole given systemically (Newman *et al.* 1989, Thomas 1990, SMTL 1999, BNF 2000). The evidence to support the use of metronidazole in malodorous wounds is limited; however, several studies and anecdotal evidence have indicated it has a deodorising ability (Thomas 1992a, Hampton 1996). The gel does not need to be reapplied daily unless the whole dressing requires changing; it can be left undisturbed for up to 2–3 days. A course of 5–7 days is recommended although re-infection is almost inevitable with chronic wounds, and treatment may need to be repeated (SMTL 1999).

Examples

Anabact®, Metrotop®*.

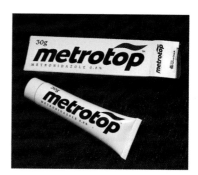

Fig. 5.10
Metronidazole gel. Reproduced from
material provided by SSL International plc.

Indications
- Malodorous fungating wounds.
- Malodorous chronic wounds (e.g. pressure ulcers, leg ulcers).

(Haughton & Young 1995)

Contra-indications
- Known hypersensitivity to metronidazole.

Precautions
- There is the possibility of systemic absorption of metronidazole and therefore systemic side effects such as nausea (Morgan 1997).

PARAFFIN GAUZE

Description
Paraffin gauze dressings consist of a fabric mesh, made from either cotton or cotton and viscose/rayon that has been impregnated with soft white or yellow paraffin (Fig. 5.11) (Morgan 1997).

Reference material
The paraffin in these dressings acts to reduce adherence of the dressing to the wound bed. It may also be known as tulle-gras.

Examples
Jelonet®, Paranet®, Paratulle®, Unitulle®*.

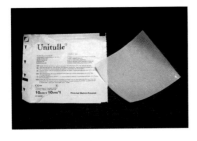

Fig. 5.11
Paraffin gauze dressing. Reproduced from material provided by Hoechst Marion Roussell.

Indications

- Superficial burns.
- Superficial ulcers.
- Split skin grafts.
- Minor traumatic injuries.

Contra-indications

- Heavily exuding wounds.
- Allergy to lanolin.

Precautions

- May dry out and adhere to the wound bed.
- May cause maceration of surrounding skin.

(Morgan 1997)

SEMI-PERMEABLE FILMS

Description

Semi-permeable film dressings usually consist of a polyurethane film with a hypoallergenic acrylic adhesive and have a variety of application methods often consisting of a plastic or cardboard carrier (Fig. 5.12) (Jones & Milton 2000a).

Reference material

These dressings are permeable to water vapour and oxygen but impermeable to micro-organisms. Permeability to water vapour varies between dressings, for

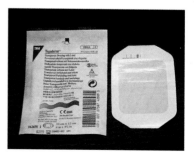

Fig. 5.12
A semi-permeable film. Reproduced from material provided by 3M Health Care Limited.

example Opsite IV3000® is highly permeable to water vapour (about $3000 g/m^2$ /24 hours) and therefore prevents the build-up of moisture beneath the dressing.

Examples
Bioclusive®, Cutifilm®, Epiview®, Opsite Flexigrid®, Opsite IV3000®*, Tegaderm®*.

Indications
- Superficial, low exudate wounds.
- Surgical wounds healing by primary intention (i.e. closed surgical wounds).
- Prevention of skin breakdown in high friction areas (sacrum, elbows, heels).
- As a retention dressing.
- Central venous catheters and long term peripheral intravenous (IV) catheters (Opsite IV3000®, Tegaderm IV®).

(Miller & Dyson 1996, Jones & Milton 2000a)

Contra-indications
- Deep cavities or third degree burns.
- Infected wounds.
- Moderate and highly exuding wounds.

(Miller & Dyson 1996, SMTL 1999)

Precautions
- Build-up of excess exudate under the dressing may cause skin maceration.
- Adhesive trauma may occur on removal from fragile skin.
- Allows cooling of the wound surface.

(Morgan 1997)

SILICONE GEL SHEETING

Description
Silicone gel sheeting is a soft, semi-occlusive sheet made from medical grade silicone (Fig. 5.13) (Williams 1996b).

Reference material
The way in which silicone gel sheeting exerts its effect is not known; however, a number of studies have shown its ability to soften, as well as reduce the size

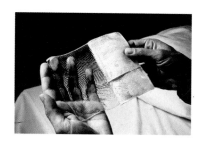

Fig. 5.13
Silicone gel sheeting. Reproduced from
material provided by Smith & Nephew
Healthcare Limited.

and colour of, hypertrophic and keloid scars (Carney *et al.* 1994, Williams 1996b). If the scar is in an awkward position, the sheeting may need extra securing with hypoallergenic tape or an elastic conforming bandage (e.g. Netelast®). The gel sheet must be removed and washed twice a day in warm water with a mild, non-oily soap and dried with paper towelling. The sheet will need to be replaced approximately every 2 weeks or if it starts to break apart or becomes difficult to fix in place (SMTL 1999). When used as a preventative measure for scar formation this product should only be applied to surgical incisions after the sutures have been removed.

Note: In order to reduce any irritation caused by the gel sheet, it is recommended that patients acclimatise their skin by slowly building up the amount of time the gel is in place. This should be done as follows: 4 h for the first 2 days, 8 h for the next two days and then increasing by 2 h per day until the sheet is being worn for 24 h. In some cases patients may not be able to tolerate having the gel sheet in place for 24 h, usually due to the development of a rash. In this instance they should wear it 12 h on and 12 h off (Carney *et al.* 1994, Williams 1996b, SMTL 1999).

Examples
Cica-Care®*, Mepiform®, Silgel®.

Indications
- Existing and new hypertrophic and keloid scars.
- Prophylactically for prevention of hypertrophic and keloid scar formation.

(SMTL 1999)

Contra-indications

- Patients with dermatological conditions causing impaired skin integrity within the area of treatment.
- Development of irritation, flaking, weeping or blistering of the skin.
- Not to be used on open wounds.

(SMTL 1999)

SKIN BARRIER FILMS

Description

These include a new generation of liquid polymer films that are alcohol-free and form a protective film on the skin (Fig. 5.14).

Reference material

These films are a replacement for many of the film dressings, ointments and creams commonly used in the protection of damaged or fragile skin. The films are non-cytotoxic and, because they do not contain alcohol, do not sting if applied to raw areas of skin (Williams 1998, Williams 1999c). When dry they form flexible protective films on the skin that have a high wash-off resistance and protect the skin from body fluids (including urine, diarrhoea, saliva and

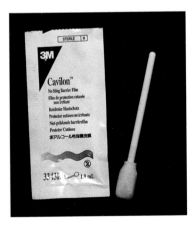

Fig. 5.14
A skin barrier film. Reproduced from material provided by 3M Health Care Limited.

wound exudate), friction and shear as well as the effects of adhesive products (Rolstad *et al.* 1994, Hampton 1998).

The two available products have different application techniques due to their presentation. Cavilon® is available in two sizes of foam applicators, 1 ml and 3 ml, that can be used to apply film to small areas of skin and are especially useful around stomas, fistulae and wounds. There is also a pump spray suitable for larger areas of skin such as the sacral area. SuperSkin® is supplied in a dropper bottle, and the liquid is spread onto the skin with a finger. For both products a single coating of the film is applied to the skin and dries in about 1 minute. Neither film needs to be removed and the film should be reapplied every 24–48 hours (Williams 1998, Williams 1999c).

Examples

Cavilon®*, SuperSkin®.

Indications

- Incontinence of both urine and faeces.
- Artificial skin openings such as fistulae, stomas and tracheostomies (particularly if the drainage from these sites is corrosive to the skin, such as that from an ileostomy).
- Wound margins to prevent maceration of the skin by exudate and to reduce skin stripping by adhesive tapes. The films also provide an excellent base for adhesives to stick to.
- Radiation induced skin reactions (have only been investigated with SuperSkin®).
- Moisture (i.e. areas that are prone to, or have become damaged by, moisture such as sweat).

(Goebel & Hazuka 1997, Williams 1998, Williams 1999c)

SUGAR PASTE

Definition

Sugar paste used in wound care is a mixture of icing sugar, caster sugar, polyethylene glycol and hydrogen peroxide combined to form either a thin or thick consistency (Morgan 1997).

Reference material

Sugar is another traditional product that has been used in wound care for many years. It has been used extensively at Northwick Park Hospital in the UK (Middleton 1990) and was recently investigated at the Royal Cornwall Hospital (Newton & Hutchings 1999). In its early application ordinary granulated sugar was used on wounds, but this can cause a severe burning sensation when applied to open wounds due to the rapid uptake of moisture by the sugar (Topham 1991). Also, granulated sugar may not be sterile and may contain anti-caking agents such as cornstarch (Addison & Walterspiel 1985). It is now common practice to use a paste, which may be made according to a recipe perfected at Northwick Park Hospital (Table 5.1).

The thin version can be used for cavity or sinus wounds with small openings while the thick paste is similar in consistency to modelling clay and can be moulded into shape and used in open cavities or more superficial wounds such as leg ulcers (Morgan 1997). Sugar paste has a high osmolarity and will compete for water in the wound, thereby preventing bacterial growth. It also reduces the wound pH to 5, which could also affect bacterial growth (Middleton 1990). Sugar paste will assist in the debridement of sloughy wounds and this action combined with its antibacterial effects will reduce wound malodour.

Indications

- Infected wounds (in particular pressure ulcers and vulval wounds).
- Malodorous wounds.
- Abscesses.
- Cavity or sinus wounds.
- Burns.

(Gordon *et al.* 1985, Dawson 1996, Morgan 1997)

Table 5.1 Recipe for thin and thick sugar pastes.

	Thin paste	Thick paste
Caster sugar	1200 g	1200 g
Icing sugar (calcium and magnesium free)	1800 g	1800 g
Polyethylene glycol 400	1416 ml	686 ml
Hydrogen peroxide 30%	23.1 ml	19 ml

(Middleton 1990, Morgan 1997)

Contra-indication

* Impaired renal function as the polyethylene glycol may be absorbed and high levels can be nephrotoxic (Middleton 1990).

TOPICAL NEGATIVE PRESSURE THERAPY

Description

Topical negative pressure therapy (also called vacuum assisted closure) involves the application of topical negative pressure uniformly across the wound surface by a vacuum device (Collier 1997, Banwell 1999).

Reference material

Topical negative pressure therapy has been shown to improve blood flow, promote formation of granulation tissue, and reduce bacterial colonisation (Morykwas *et al.* 1997). Negative pressure therapy may be used in plastic surgery to promote formation of granulation tissue and avoid the need for a free flap, or it may be used to secure split thickness skin grafts in place (Argenta & Morykwas 1997, Schneider *et al.* 1998, Banwell 1999).

An example of a device available in the UK that can be used to deliver topical negative pressure therapy is the VAC® (Vacuum Assisted Closure) Wound Closure System (Fig. 5.15). This is a commercially available device that has the ability to deliver either continuous or intermittent negative pressure. The system comes with a sterile open pore foam sponge that has a fenestrated drainage tube inserted into it, a cartridge and connection tubing and the negative pressure pump. It is also available as a 'Mini VAC®' that fits into a small pouch which

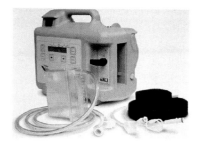

Fig. 5.15
The VAC topical negative pressure device (photograph kindly supplied by KCI Medical Ltd). Reproduced with permission from KCI.

can be worn over the shoulder or as a 'bum-bag'. This is battery powered so patients can remain mobile and receive treatment at home.

The sterile foam sponge is cut to the shape of the wound and then sterile suction tubing is inserted into the sponge, which is then placed on or into the wound. This is covered with an occlusive dressing to form a seal around the wound and the suction tubing is attached to the VAC unit (Mendez-Eastman 1998). The foam dressing is usually left in place for 2 days, except in the case of SSGs. The plastic surgeon will stipulate the frequency of dressing renewal and will specify the type of pressure required, e.g. intermittent or continuous. A negative pressure of 50 to 75 mmHg is generally used to secure SSGs, while a range of 50 to 200 mmHg may be used for open wounds, with 125 mmHg being the usual negative pressure utilised (Baxandall 1997, Banwell 1999). The in-growth of granulation tissue into the foam is a common occurrence but this can be avoided by using a non-adherent dressing such as a silicone coated polyamide net (Mepitel®) to line the wound bed (Banwell 1999).

When the machine is switched on, a uniform vacuum is created across the wound, evident from the crinkling effect of the foam. This negative pressure removes excess tissue fluid, thereby reducing oedema and preventing exudate build-up. In addition, the negative pressure causes dilation of arterioles hence improving local blood circulation and increasing the supply of oxygen and nutrients to the wound (Morykwas *et al.* 1997). This promotes the formation of granulation tissue and speeds wound closure (Argenta & Morykwas 1997). The traction on the cells by the negative pressure is also thought to promote cell division within the wound (Mendez-Eastman 1998).

Aerobic bacteria in the wound are starved of oxygen in the negative pressure environment and, coupled with the removal of exudate and sloughy tissue, this reduces the bacterial load on the wound (Hampton 1999b).

Indications

Topical negative pressure therapy can be used on both acute and chronic wounds including:

- Venous and diabetic ulcers.
- Pressure ulcers.
- Surgical flaps.

- Dehisced surgical wounds.
- Fixation of meshed SSGs.

> (Argenta & Morykwas 1997, Collier 1997, Morykwas & Argenta 1997)

Contra-indications

- Fistulae.
- Any wound that contains dry necrotic tissue.
- Malignancy.
- Actively bleeding wounds.
- Patients taking anticoagulants.

> (Collier 1997)

SECONDARY DRESSINGS

Definition

A secondary dressing overlies the primary wound contact dressing and is not in direct contact with the wound bed.

Reference material

Secondary dressings may include low-linting gauze squares, absorbent pads, cotton wool and bandages (Thomas 1998). These perform a number of functions depending on the type chosen. The main points governing the choice of secondary dressing are the amount of exudate being produced by the wound and the choice of primary dressing.

Examples

Low-linting gauze squares, orthopaedic wadding bandages, Sugripad®*.

Indications

- Holding a primary dressing in place.
- Providing extra absorbency.
- Providing extra protection from infection and trauma.
- Retaining moisture in low exuding, or dry wounds.
- Containment of malodour.

> (Thomas 1998)

TAPES

Definition
There are a large variety of tapes available. They may be made from plastic, paper or fabric and use a range of adhesive substances.

Reference material
Tapes are used to retain dressings, bandages or other medical appliances in position. When used to secure dressings, tapes should be hypoallergenic and only fixed to healthy normal skin, as they may cause trauma upon removal from fragile or diseased skin. Dressings should be large enough to extend over the whole wound and onto healthy skin to allow for this.

For patients with very sensitive and/or diseased skin, or with an allergy to adhesives, tape should be avoided on the skin surrounding a wound. In the case of unhealthy or diseased skin (very commonly seen in malignant wounds where disease is invading surrounding skin), plain bandaging or elastic conforming bandages should be used to secure dressings.

Examples
Netelast®*, Tubifast®.

The following points can be used as a guide to choosing tapes:

(1) Sensitive skin
- Hypoallergenic tape is a suitable choice for most dressings.

Examples
Micropore®*, Blenderm®*.

(2) Dressing over an area subject to movement, for example joints
- Hypoallergenic tapes that are flexible and/or elastic (these tapes are also waterproof).

Example
Transpore®*.

(3) Large or heavy dressings and for securing catheters and drainage tubing
- Retention sheets (larger fabric tapes) are a good choice to hold heavy, bulky dressings in place (SMTL 1999)

Examples
Mefix®*, Hypafix®.

Care should be taken to ensure tapes are applied correctly. If the tape is applied under tension the skin will 'ruck up' underneath and blistering may occur (SMTL 1999).

WOUND MANAGEMENT PRODUCTS TO BE AVOIDED OR FOR RESTRICTED USE ONLY

There are a number of conflicting views concerning the use of the products listed below which have traditionally been used for wound management (Harding 1996, Lawrence 1996, Moore 1996). Many of them have been shown to be either ineffective, damaging to wound tissues and/or to delay healing (Brennan & Leaper 1985). In the interests of patient and staff safety, the products are listed in Table 5.2 and are not recommended for routine use.

Table 5.2 outlines the problems, and potential adverse effects, of using these products. The specific instances where these products may be used are also indicated. However, there is often an alternative, safer, more effective product that may be selected in their place.

Use of topical antiseptics and antibiotics

The use of antiseptic solutions in wound management is still very controversial. Most authors agree that their use should be restricted, if not abandoned, due to their toxic effects on healthy tissue and the fact that they are rapidly inactivated on contact with organic matter (Tatnall *et al.* 1990, Leaper 1996, Trevelyn 1996, Fletcher 1997, Oliver 1997, Gilchrist 1999). Opinion is also divided on the use of topical antibiotics. They may lead to the development of bacterial resistance to systemic antibiotics and skin sensitivity reactions (Thomas 1990, Thomas 1997, Miller 1998b, Gilchrist 1999). Exceptions are:

(1) Silver sulphadiazine cream for the prevention of infection in burns and for the treatment of infected skin graft donor sites.

Table 5.2 Products to be avoided or for 'restricted use' in wound management.

Product	Reasons for avoidance	Restricted uses
Cetrimide products	Toxic to fibroblasts May develop skin irritation and sensitisation Stored product may become contaminated by *Pseudomonas* (Leaper 1996, Miller & Dyson 1996, Trevelyn 1996)	Use with caution in infected or heavily contaminated wounds only
Chlorhexidine products	Toxic to cells Ineffective against some strains of MRSA Potential for sensitivity and anaphylactic reactions Stored product may become contaminated by *Pseudomonas* (Tatnall *et al.* 1990, Miller & Dyson 1996)	Use restricted to skin cleansing only
Cicatrin powder	May cause systemic side effects, hypersensitivity reaction or contact dermatitis Forms a 'cake' in wounds that may cause irritation (Morgan 1997)	Not recommended for use on open wounds
Eusol (sodium hypochlorite solution)	Limited debriding ability Toxic to healing tissue Rapidly deactivated by organic material, blood, pus and exudate (Catlin 1992, Lawrence 1996, Oliver 1997, Gilchrist 1999)	Generally not recommended for use in open wounds but may be used for only a short period, in heavily infected wounds (Leaper 1996, Miller 1998b)
Fusidic acid (Fucidin)	Narrow-spectrum antibiotic for use with penicillin-resistant staphylococci Risk of skin sensitisation (Morgan 1997, BNF 2000)	Not recommended for use on open wounds

Table 5.2 *Continued*

Product	Reasons for avoidance	Restricted uses
Gentian violet (crystal violet)	Possibly carcinogenic (evidence in animals) (Aidoo *et al.* 1990, Murphy 1995) Causes staining and is messy to use	Avoid use in open wounds
Hydrogen peroxide	Deactivated by organic material such as pus and wound exudate May be caustic to surrounding skin Danger of embolus formation if used in closed body cavities or under pressure (Sleigh & Linter 1985, Murphy 1995, Miller & Dyson 1996, Trevelyn 1996, Hampton 1999a)	May be used in superficial, heavily contaminated traumatic wounds e.g. from a road traffic accident
Low-linting gauze (as primary dressing)	Danger of adherence and shedding of fibres into wound Incorporates into granulation tissue and therefore damages tissues on removal (Johnson 1988b, Miller & Dyson 1996)	Not recommended for use as a primary dressing on open wounds
Milton solution	Disinfectant solution (sodium hypochlorite) (see Eusol).	Not recommended for use on open wounds
Mupirocin (Bactroban)	Stinging, burning or itching may occur on application (Trevelyn 1996, Miller 1998b)	Used for bacterial skin infections Possible use in wounds infected by MRSA Only use after advice from consultant microbiologist
Phenoxytol	Toxicity not well researched Active against *Pseudomonas aeruginosa* (Morgan 1997)	Use restricted to skin cleansing

Table 5.2 *Continued*

Product	Reasons for avoidance	Restricted uses
Povidone iodine products	Toxic to fibroblasts Deactivated by organic material Danger of systemic absorption and allergic dermatitis (Cameron & Leaper 1988, Miller & Dyson 1996)	Use of povidone iodine solution restricted to skin cleansing only at present Recent studies have suggested that certain forms of iodine may be useful for infected wounds, for example as cadexomer beads. (Oliver 1997, Miller 1998b, Gilchrist 1999, Gulliver 1999)
Proflavine cream	Slow acting antiseptic Mildly bacteriostatic against gram positive organisms Contains lanolin, which may cause skin hypersensitivity reactions May stain clothing (SMTL 1995, Morgan 1997) Causes gene mutation in some viral, bacterial and mammalian cell lines. Possible carcinogenic risk (IARC 1998)	Used for minor cuts and burns and as a second line treatment in moist desquamation reactions to radiotherapy
Silver sulphadiazine (Flamazine®)	Potential for sensitivity reaction and argyria (slate grey discoloration of the skin due to silver deposition) Potential side effect of leucopenia has been noted with excessive use (Leaper 1996, Morgan 1997, BNF 2000)	Use restricted for prophylaxis of infection in burns, skin graft donor sites and GvHD

Table 5.2 *Continued*

Product	Reasons for avoidance	Restricted uses
Terra-Cortril (oxytetracycline + hydrocortisone)	Topical antibiotic and steroid, which are not recommended for use on open wounds	Used for treating hypergranulation tissue under direction from a plastic surgeon. Use sparingly and only for a short period (Morgan 1997)

(2) Metronidazole gel for deodorising chronic wounds.
(3) Mupirocin for wounds infected with MRSA (seek advice from consultant microbiologist before use).

(Leaper 1996, Trevelyn 1996, Morgan 1997, Miller 1998b)

Antibiotic treatment is only required when there is overt clinical infection (see section on infected wounds in Chapter 3) and in this situation systemic therapy should be initiated. There is no substitute for good aseptic technique and the correct use of occlusive dressings to minimise the risk of wound infection.

CONCLUSION

This chapter has summarised the many wound management products available to health care professionals. However, the range and number of products is constantly changing and it is the practitioner's responsibility to remain up-to-date with the latest technology. It is also vital that practitioners are aware of current research into the efficacy of wound management products. Practitioners are reminded that the selection of these products should only occur after a thorough assessment to ensure that they will meet desired outcomes stated in the wound management care plan.

References

Adam, K. & Oswald, I. (1983) Protein synthesis, bodily renewal and the sleep-wake cycle. *Clinical Science*, **65**(6), 561–7.

Adams, J. F. & Lassen, L. F. (1995) Leech therapy for venous congestion following myocutaneous pectoralis flap reconstruction. *ORL – Head and Neck Nursing*, **13**(1), 12–14.

Addison, M. K. & Walterspiel, J. N. (1985) Sugar and wound healing (letter). *The Lancet*, **2**(8456), 665.

Aidoo, A., Gao, N., Neft, R. E., Schol, H. M., Hass, B. S., Minor, T. Y. & Heflich, R. H. (1990) Evaluation of the genotoxicity of gentian violet in bacterial and mammalian cell systems. *Teratog Carcinog Mutagen*, **10**(6), 449–62.

Alfaro-Lefevre, R. (1999) *Critical Thinking in Nursing: A Practical Approach*, 2nd edn. W.B. Saunders, Philidelphia.

Allsworth, J. (1985) *Skin Camouflage. A Guide to Remedial Techniques*. Arnold-Taylor Education Ltd, London.

Aractingi, S. & Chosidow, O. (1998) Cutaneous graft-versus-host disease. *Archives of Dermatology*, **134**, 602–12.

Argenta, L. C. & Morykwas, M. J. (1997) Vacuum-assisted closure: a new method for wound control and treatment: clinical experience. *Annals of Plastic Surgery*, **38**(6), 563–76.

Armstrong, M. (1998) Obesity as an intrinsic factor affecting wound healing. *Journal of Wound Care*, **7**(5), 220–21.

Ashford, R., Plant, G., Maher, J. & Teares, L. (1980) Metronidazole in smelly tumours. *Lancet*, **1**(1), 874–5.

Bachand, P. M. & McNicholas, M. E. (1999) Creating a wound assessment chart. *Advances in Wound Care*, **12**, 426–9.

Back, I. N. & Finlay, I. (1995) Analgesic effect of topical opioids on painful skin ulcers (Letter). *Journal of Pain and Symptom Management*, **10**(7), 493.

Baker, P. G. & Haig, G. (1981) Metronidazole in the treatment of chronic pressure sores and ulcers: a comparison with standard treatments in general practice. *The Practitioner*, **225**, 569–73.

Balakrishnan, C. (1994) Simple method of applying pressure to skin grafts of neck with foam dressing and staples. *Journal of Burn Care and Rehabilitation*, **15**(5), 432–3.

Bale, S. (1997) A guide to wound debridement. *Journal of Wound Care*, **6**(4), 179–82.

Bale, S. & Collier, M. (1998) *Cavity wounds.* Educational Leaflet 5(1) revised. The Wound Care Society, Huntingdon, UK.

Bale, S. & Harding, K. G. (1991) Foams still find favour: wound management using foam dressings. *Professional Nurse*, June, 510–18.

Bale, S. & Jones, V. (1997) *Wound Care Nursing A Patient-Centred Approach.* Baillière Tindall, London.

Banwell, P. E. (1999) Topical negative pressure therapy in wound care. *Journal of Wound Care*, **8**(2), 79–84.

Barkham, A. M. (1993) Radiotherapy skin reactions and treatments. *Professional Nurse*, **8**, 732–6.

Baum, T. M. & Busuito, M. J. (1997) Use of a glycerin-based gel sheeting in scar management. *Advances in Wound Care*, **11**(1), 40–43.

Baxandall, T. (1997) Healing cavity wounds with negative pressure. *Elderly Care*, **9**(1), 20–22.

Benbow, M. (1995) Parameters of wound assessment. *British Journal of Nursing*, **4**(11), 647–51.

Bennett, G. & Moody, M. (1995) *Wound Care for Health Professionals.* Chapman and Hall, London.

Berry, D. & Jones, V. (1993) Cavity wound management. *Journal of Wound Care*, **2**(1), 29–32.

Bertin, M. L., Crowe, J. & Gordon, S. M. (1998) Determinants of surgical site infection after breast surgery. *American Journal of Infection Control*, **26**(1), 61–5.

Biopharm (1996) *Clinical Use of Leeches*, (Online), available from URL: http://www.biopharm-leeches.com/uses.htm, (accessed 19 July 2000).

Biopharm (1998) *Caution Contra-indication for the Leech Arterial Insufficiency*, (Online), available from URL: http://www.biopharm-leeches.com/caution.htm, (accessed 19 July 2000).

Biopharm (1999) *Leech Maintenance*, (Online), available from URL: http://www.biopharm-leeches.com/maint.htm, (accessed 19 July 2000).

Biosurgical Research Unit (1999) *Data Card Larv E Version 2.1.* Biosurgical Research Unit, Princes of Wales Hospital, Bridgend.

Bird, C. (2000) Supporting patients with fungating breast wounds. *Professional Nurse*, **15**(10), 649–52.

Blackmar, A. (1997) Focus on wound care: radiation-induced skin alterations. *MEDSURG Nursing*, **6**(3), 172–5.

Bland, K. I., Palin, W. E., van Fraunhofer, A., Morris, R. R., Adcock, R. A. & Tobin, G. R. (1984) Experimental and clinical observations of the effects of cytotoxic chemotherapeutic drugs on wound healing. *Annals of Surgery*, **199**(6), 782–9.

References

BNF (2000) *British National Formulary* Number 39 (March). British Medical Association and the Royal Pharmaceutical Society of Great Britain, London.

Boot-Vickers, M. & Eaton, K. (1999) Skin care for patients receiving radiotherapy. *Professional Nurse*, **14**(10), 706–708.

Bower, M., Stein, R., Evans, T. R. J., Hedley, A., Pert, P. & Coombes, R. C. (1992) A double-blind study of the efficacy of metronidazole gel in the treatment of malodorous fungating tumours. *European Journal of Cancer*, **28a**(4/5), 888–9.

Bowler, P. (1998) The anaerobic and aerobic microbiology of wounds: a review. *Wounds*, **10**(6), 170–78.

Bradley, M., Cullum, N. & Sheldon T. (1999) The debridement of chronic wounds: a systematic review. *Health Technology Assessment*, **3**(17) (Pt 1). The National Coordinating Centre for Health Technology Assessment, Southampton, UK.

Brennan, S. S. & Leaper, D. J. (1985) The effect of antiseptics on the healing wound: a study using the rabbit ear chamber. *British Journal of Surgery*, **72**, 780–82.

Briggs, M., Wilson, S. & Fuller, A. (1996) The principles of aseptic technique in wound care. *Professional Nurse*, **11**(12), 805–808.

Brown, A. S., Glickman, L. T., Matthews, M. S. & Slezak, S. (1998) *Essentials for Students – Plastic and Reconstructive Surgery*, (Online), 5th edn, Plastic Surgery Information Service, available from URL: http://www.plasticsurgery.org/profinfo/essen/essentials.htm (accessed 17 October 1999).

Buchsel, P. C. (1997) Allogenic bone marrow transplantation. In: *Cancer Nursing. Principles and Practice*, 4th edn (eds S. L. Groenwald, M. Hansen Frogge, M. Goodman & C. Henke Yarbro), pp. 459–506. Jones and Bartlett Publishers, Boston.

Calvin, M. (1998) Cutaneous wound repair. *Wounds*, **10**(1), 12–32.

Cameron, S. & Leaper, D. (1988) Antiseptic toxicity in open wounds. *Nursing Times*, **84**(25), 77–9.

Campbell, I. R. & Illingworth, M. H. (1992) Can patients wash during radiotherapy to the breast or chest wall? A randomized controlled trial. *Clinical Oncology*, **4**, 78–82.

Campbell, J. & Lane, C. (1996) Developing a skin-care protocol in radiotherapy. *Professional Nurse*, **12**(2), 105–108.

Capra, L. (1986) *The Care of the Cancer Patient*. Macmillan Magazines Ltd, London.

Carney, S. A., Cason, C. G., Gowar, J. P., Stevenson, J. H., McNee, J., Groves, A. R., Thomas, S. S., Hart, N. B. & Auclair, P. (1994) Cica-care gel sheeting in the management of hypertrophic scarring. *Burns*, **20**(2), 163–7.

Casey, G. (1997) Assessing wounds. *Kai-Tiaki: Nursing New Zealand*, **3**(5), 26.

Casey, G. (1998) The management of pain in wound care. *Nursing Standard*, **13**(12), 49–54.

Catlin, L. (1992) The use of hypochlorite solutions in wound management. *British Journal of Nursing*, **1**(5), 226–9.

Clamon, J. & Netscher, D. T. (1994) General principles of flap reconstruction: goals for aesthetic and functional outcome. *Plastic Surgical Nursing*, **14**(1), 9–14.

Collier, M. (1994) Assessing a wound. *Nursing Standard* 8(49). RCN Nursing Update 3–8.

Collier, M. (1996) The principles of optimum wound management. *Nursing Standard*, **10**(43), 47–52.

Collier, M. (1997) Know how: vacuum-assisted closure (VAC). *Nursing Times*, **93**(5), 32–5.

Collinson, G. (1992) Improving quality of life in patients with malignant fungating wounds. *Second European Conference on Advances in Wound Management (proceedings)*, pp. 59–61. Macmillan Magazines Ltd, London.

Cooper, D. (1993) Managing malignant ulcers effectively. *Nursing Standard*, **8**(2), 25–8.

Cooper, R. & Molan, P. (1999) The role of honey as an antiseptic in managing *Pseudomonas* infection. *Journal of Wound Care*, **8**(4), 161–4.

Copp, K. (1991) Nursing patients having radiotherapy. In: *Oncology for Nurses and Health Care Professionals, Vol. 3, Cancer Nursing*, 2nd edn (eds R. Tiffany & D. Borley), pp. 38–73. HarperCollins Academic, London.

Coull, A. (1991) Making Sense of . . . Split Skin Grafts. *Nursing Times*, **87**(27), 54–5.

Coull, A. (1992) Making Sense of . . . Surgical Flaps. *Nursing Times*, **88**(1), 32–34.

Coull, A. & Wylie, K. (1990) Regular monitoring: the way to ensure flap healing. *Professional Nurse*, October, 18–21.

Coull, A. F. (1993) Using leeches for venous drainage after surgery. *Journal of Wound Care*, **2**(5), 294–7.

Cruse, P. J. E. & Ford, R. (1980) The epidemiology of wound infections; a ten year prospective study of 62939 wounds. *Surgical Clinics of North America*, **60**, 27–40.

Cutting, K. (1994) Factors affecting wound healing. *Nursing Standard*, **8**(50), 33–6.

Cutting, K. F. (1998) *Wounds and infection*. Educational Leaflet 5(2). The Wound Care Society, Huntingdon, UK.

Cutting, K. (1999) Glossary. In: *Wound Management Theory and Practice* (eds M. Miller & D. Glover), pp. 170–73. Nursing Times Books, London.

Danton, S. (1987) Fashionable blood suckers. *Nursing Times*, **83**(5), 53–4.

Davies, D. M. (1985a) Plastic and reconstructive surgery: scars, hypertrophic scars and keloids. *British Medical Journal*, **290**(6474), 1056–58.

Davies, D. M. (1985b) Plastic and reconstructive surgery: skin cover. *British Medical Journal*, **290**(6470), 765–8.

Dawson, C., Armstrong, M. W., Fulford, S. C., Faruqi, R. M. & Galland, R. B. (1992) Use of calcium alginate to pack abscess cavities: a controlled clinical trial. *Journal of the Royal College of Surgeons Edinburgh*, **37**(3), 177–9.

Dawson, J. S. (1996) The role of sugar in wound healing. *Annals of the Royal College of Surgeons England*, **78**(2) Suppl, 82–5.

Dealey, C. (1999) *The Care of Wounds*. 2nd edn. Blackwell Science, Oxford.

DeMeyer, E. S., Fletcher, M. A. & Buschel, P. (1997) Management of dermatologic complications of chronic graft versus host disease: a case study. *Clinical Journal of Oncology Nursing*, **1**(4), 95–104.

DoH (1998) *Review of Prescribing, Supply and Administration of Medicines: a Report on the Supply and Administration of Medicines Under Group Protocols*. Department of Health, Stationery Office, London.

DoH (1999) *Review of Prescribing, Supply and Administration of Medicines, Final Report*. Department of Health, Stationery Office, London.

Dougherty, L., Mallett, J. & Root, T. (2000) Drug administration. In: *The Royal Marsden Hospital Manual of Clinical Nursing Procedures*, 5th edn (eds J. Mallett & L. Dougherty), pp. 211–54, Blackwell Science, Oxford.

Dunford, C. (1997) Know how: management of cavity wounds. *Nursing Times*, **93**(32), 72–3.

Dyson, M., Young, S., Pendle, C. L., Webster, D. F. & Lang, S. M. (1988) Comparison of the effects of moist and dry conditions on dermal repair. *Journal of Investigative Dermatology*, **91**, 434–9.

Dyson, M., Young, S. R., Hart, J., Lynch, J. A. & Lang, S. (1992) Comparison of the effects of moist and dry conditions on the process of angiogenesis during dermal repair. *Journal of Investigative Dermatology*, **99**, 729–33.

Eaglstein, W. H. (1985) The effect of occlusive dressings on collagen synthesis and re-epithelialization in superficial wounds. In: *An Environment for Healing: The Role of Occlusion*. Royal Society of Medicine International Congress and Symposium Series No. 88. (ed. T. J. Ryan), pp. 31–4. Royal Society of Medicine, London.

Edwards, K. (1994) Skin flaps in plastic surgery: an overview. *Nursing Standard*, **9**(4), 27–30.

Ehrenberg, A., Ehnfors, M. & Thorell-Ekstrand, I. (1996) Nursing documentation in patient records: experience of the use of the VIPS model. *Journal of Advanced Nursing*, **24**, 853–67.

Ehrlich, H. P. (1999) The physiology of wound healing: a summary of normal and abnormal wound healing processes. *Advances in Wound Care*, (Online), available from URL: http://www.woundcarenet.com/advances/articles/woundhealing.htm (accessed 3 July 2000).

Eisenbeiss, W., Peter, F. W., Bakhtiari, C. & Frenz, C. (1998) Hypertrophic scars and keloids. *Journal of Wound Care*, **7**(5), 255–7.

Emflorgo, C. (1998) Controlling bleeding in fungating wounds (letter). *Journal of Wound Care*, **7**(5), 235.

Everrett, W. G. (1985) Wound sinus or fistula. In *Wound Care* (ed. S. Westaby), pp. 84–90. Heinemann Medical Books Ltd, London.

Finlay, I., Bowszyc, J., Ramlau, C. & Gwiezdzinski, Z. (1996) The effect of 0.75% metronidazole gel on malodorous cutaneous ulcers. *Journal of Pain and Symptom Management*, **11**(3), 158–62.

Flanagan, M. (1994) Assessment criteria. *Nursing Times*, **90**(35), 76–88.

Flanagan, M. (1996) A practical framework for wound assessment 1: physiology. *British Journal of Nursing*, **5**(22), 1391–7.

Flanagan, M. (1997) A practical framework for wound assessment 2: methods. *British Journal of Nursing*, **6**(1), 6–11.

Flanagan, M. (1998) The characteristics and formation of granulation tissue. *Journal of Wound Care*, **7**(10), 508–10.

Flanagan, M. (1999) The physiology of wound healing. In: *Wound Management Theory and Practice*, (eds M. Miller & D. Glover), pp. 14–22. Nursing Times Books, London.

Flanagan, M. (2000) The physiology of wound healing. *Journal of Wound Care*, **9**(6), 299–300.

Fletcher, J. (1997) Update: wound cleansing. *Professional Nurse*, **12**(11), 793–6.

Fletcher, J. (2000) The role of collagen in wound healing. *Professional Nurse*, **15**(8), 527–30.

Forbes, A. & Myers, C. (1996) Enterocutaneous fistulae and their management. In: *Stoma Care Nursing a Patient-Centred Approach* (ed. C. Myers), pp. 63–77. Arnold, London.

Foster, L. & Moore, P. (1998) Acute surgical wound care 3: fitting the dressing to the wound. *British Journal of Nursing*, **8**(4), 200–10.

Francis, A. (1998) Nursing management of skin graft sites. *Nursing Standard*, **12**(33), 41–4.

Freedline, A. (1999) *Types of wound debridement* (Online). The Wound Care Information Network, available from URL: http://www.medicaledu.com/debridhp.htm (accessed 8 October 1999).

Gacheru, I. (1998) Maggots in the treatment of necrotising faciitis. *The Nairobi Hospital Proceedings*, **2**(4), 234–8.

Galvani, J. (1997) Not yet cut and dried. *Nursing Times*, **93**(16), 88–9.

Garrett, B. (1997) The proliferation and movement of cells during re-epithelialisation. *Journal of Wound Care*, **6**(4), 174–7.

Gelbart, M. (1999) Wounds in time: the history of wound management. In: *Wound Management Theory and Practice*, (eds M. Miller & D. Glover), pp. 1–13. Nursing Times Books, London.

Gibson, B. (1995) *A Cost Effectiveness Comparison of Two Gels in the Treatment of Sloughy Leg Ulcers.* Presented at the Advanced Wound Care Symposium, San Diego.

Gilchrist, B. (1999) Wound infection. In: *Wound Management Theory and Practice*, (eds M. Miller & D. Glover), pp. 96–106. Nursing Times Books, London.

Goebel, R. H. & Hazuka, M. B. (1997) *Prevention of radiation-induced dermatitis by superskin, a polymer adhesive skin sealant*. Available from Medlogic Global Ltd, Plymouth.

Goodman, M., Hilderley, L. J. & Purl, S. (1997) Integumentary and mucous membrane alterations. In: *Cancer Nursing. Principles and Practice*, 4th edn, (eds S. L. Groenwald, M. Hansen Frogge, M. Goodman & C. Henke Yarbro), pp. 768–822, Jones and Bartlett Publishers, Boston.

Gordon, H., Middleton, K., Seal, D. & Sullens, K. (1985) Sugar and wound healing (letter). *The Lancet*, **2**(8456), 663–4.

Gordon, M. (1994) *Nursing Diagnosis, Process and Application*. Mosby, Missouri.

Grocott, P. (1995) The palliative management of fungating malignant wounds. *Journal of Wound Care*, **4**(5), 240–42.

Grocott, P. (1998) Exudate management in fungating wounds. *Journal of Wound Care*, **7**(9), 445–8.

Grocott, P. (2000) The palliative management of fungating malignant wounds. *Journal of Wound Care*, **9**(1), 4–9.

Gulliver, G. (1999) Arguments over iodine. *Nursing Times*, **95**(27), 68–70.

Haisfield-Wolfe, M. E. & Baxendale-Cox, L. M. (1999) Staging of malignant cutaneous wounds: a pilot study. *Oncology Nursing Forum*, **26**(6), 1055–64.

Haisfield-Wolfe, M. E. & Rund, C. (1997) Malignant cutaneous wounds: a management protocol. *Ostomy/Wound Management*, **43**(1), 56–66.

Hallett, A. (1995a) Cavity-wound management. *Nursing Times*, **91**(30), 72,74,79.

Hallett, A. (1995b) Fungating wounds. *Nursing Times*, **91**(39), 81–5.

Hallett, A. & Hampton, S. (1999) *Wound dressings*. Educational Leaflet 6(1). The Wound Care Society, Huntingdon, UK.

Hamilton-Miller, J. M. T., Shah, S. & Smith, C. (1993) Silver sulphadiazine: a comprehensive in-vitro reassessment. *Chemotherapy*, **39**, 405–409.

Hampton, J. P. (1996) The use of metronidazole in the treatment of malodorous wounds. *Journal of Wound Care*, **5**(9), 421–6.

Hampton, S. (1998) Film subjects win the day. *Nursing Times*, **94**(24), 80–82.

Hampton, S. (1999a) Choosing the right dressing. In: *Wound Management: Theory and Practice*, (eds M. Miller & D. Glover), pp. 116–28. Nursing Times Books, London.

Hampton, S. (1999b) Wound care: vacuum wrapped. *Nursing Times*, **95**(3), 77–8.

Harding, K. G. (1996) The use of antiseptics in wound care, critique II. *Journal of Wound Care*, **5**(1), 45–6.

Hart, S (2000) Barrier nursing: nursing the infectious or immunosuppressed patient.

In: *The Royal Marsden Hospital Manual of Clinical Nursing Procedures*, 5th edn (eds J. Mallett & L. Dougherty), pp. 47–122. Blackwell Science, Oxford.

Haskins, N. (1998) Intensive nursing care of patients with a microvascular free flap after maxillofacial surgery. *Intensive & Critical Care Nursing*, **14**, 225–30.

Haughton, W. & Young, T. (1995) Common problems in wound care: malodorous wounds. *British Journal of Nursing*, **4**(16), 959–63.

Heenan, A. (1998) Frequently asked questions: alginate dressings. *World Wide Wounds* (Online), available from URL: http://www.smtl.co.uk/World-Wide-Wounds/1998/june/Alginates-FAQ/alginates-questions.html (accessed 6 October 1999).

Heenan, A. (2000) *Tariff Dressings – September 2000* (Online), Nursing Times Net, available from URL: http://www.nursingtimes.net/features/fipage.asp?story=nt20000906f01&gutter=features index gutter (accessed 21 September 2000).

Hilderley, L. J. (1997) Radiotherapy. In: *Cancer Nursing Principles and Practice*, 4th edn, (eds S. L. Groenwald, M. Hansen Frogge, M. Goodman & C. Henke Yarbro), pp. 247–82. Jones and Bartlett Publishers, Boston.

Hofman, D. (1996) Know how: A guide to wound debridement. *Nursing Times*, **92**(32), 22–3.

Hollinworth, H. (1997) Wound care – less pain, more gain. *Nursing Times*, **93**(46), 89–91.

Hopewell, J. W. (1990) The skin: its structure and response to ionizing radiation. *International Journal of Radiation Biology*, **57**(4), 751–73.

Hutchinson, J. J. & Lawrence, J. C. (1991) Wound infection under occlusive dressings. *Journal of Hospital Infection*, **17**(2), 83–94.

IARC (1998) *Proflavine, Proflavine Dihydrochloride, Proflavine Hemisulphate and Proflavine Monohydrochloride* (Online), International Agency for Research on Cancer, Lyon, France. Available from URL: http://193.51.164.11/htdocs/Monographs/Vol24/Proflavin.html, (Accessed 7 July 2000).

Irving, M. & Beadle, C. H. (1982) External intestinal fistulae: nursing care and surgical procedures. *Clinics in Gastroenterolgy*, **11**, 327–36.

Ivetić, O. & Lyne, P. A. (1990) Fungating and ulcerating malignant lesions: a review of the literature. *Journal of Advanced Nursing*, **15**, 83–8.

Jash, D. K. (1973) Epistaxis: topical use of aminocapoic acid in its management. *Journal of Laryngology and Otology*, **87**, 895–8.

Johnson & Johnson Medical (2000) *Tielle Plus Hydropolymer Adhesive Dressing* (product information). Available from: Johnson & Johnson Medical, Coronation Road, Ascot.

Johnson, A. (1988a) Natural healing process: an essential update. *The Professional Nurse*, February, 149–52.

References

Johnson, A. (1988b) Standard protocols for treating open wounds. *The Professional Nurse*, September, 498–501.

Johnson, P. A., Fleming, K. & Avery, C. M. E. (1998) Latex foam and staple fixation of skin grafts. *British Journal of Oral and Maxillofacial Surgery*, **36**, 141–2.

Jones, M., Andrews, A. & Thomas, S. (1998a) A case history describing the use of sterile larvae (maggots) in a malignant wound. *World Wide Wounds* (Online), available from URL: http://www.smtl.co.uk/World-Wide-Wounds/1998/february/ Larvae-Case-Study-Malignant-Wounds/Larvae-Case-Study-Malignant-Wounds.html (accessed 23 June 2000).

Jones, M., Davey, J. & Champion, A. (1998b) Dressing wounds. *Nursing Standard*, **12**(39), 47–52.

Jones, V. & Milton, T. (2000a) When and how to use adhesive film dressings. *Nursing Times*, **96**(14), NTPlus 3–4.

Jones, V. & Milton, T. (2000b) When and how to use hydrocolloid dressings. *Nursing Times*, **96**(4), NTPlus 5–7.

Jones, V. & Milton, T. (2000c) When and how to use hydrogels. *Nursing Times*, **96**(23), NTPlus 3–4.

Kernoble, D. S. & Kaiser, A. B. (1995) Post operative infections and antimicrobial prophylaxis. In: *Principles and Practices of Infectious Disease*, 4th edn, (eds G. L. Mandell, J. E. Bennett & R. Dolin), pp. 2742–55. Churchill Livingstone, New York.

Kiecolt-Glaser, J. K., Marucha, P. T., Malarkey, W. B., Mercado, A. M. & Glaser, R. (1995) Slowing of wound healing by psychological stress. *The Lancet*, **346**(4), 1194–6.

Lauri, S., Lepisto, M. & Kappeli, S. (1997) Patients' needs in hospital: nurses' and patients' views. *Journal of Advanced Nursing*, **25**, 339–46.

Laverty, D., Mallett, J. & Mulholland, J. (1997) Protocols and guidelines for managing wounds. *Professional Nurse*, **13**(2), 79–81.

Laverty, D., Cooper, J. & Soady, S. (2000a) Wound Management. In: *The Royal Marsden Hospital Manual of Clinical Nursing Procedures*, 5th edn (eds J. Mallett & L. Dougherty), pp. 681–710. Blackwell Science, Oxford.

Laverty, D., Naylor, W., Mallett, J. & Mulholland, J. (eds) (2000b) *The Royal Marsden Hospital Wound Management Guidelines*. Available from The Royal Marsden Hospital, London.

Lavery, B. A. (1995) Skin care during radiotherapy: a survey of UK practice. *Clinical Oncology*, **7**, 184–7.

Lawrence, J. C. (1996) The use of antiseptics in wound care, critique I. *Journal of Wound Care*, **5**(1), 44–5.

Leaper, D. (1996) Antiseptics in wound healing. *Nursing Times*, **92**(39), 63–8.

Leih, P. & Salentijn, C. (1994) Nursing diagnosis: a Dutch perspective. *Journal of Clinical Nursing*, **3**, 313–20.

Lister, A. (1991) Care of patients with malignant wounds. *Wound Management*, **3**(3), 13–15.

Lotti, T., Rodofili, C., Benci, M. & Menchin, G. (1998) Wound-healing problems associated with cancers. *Journal of Wound Care*, **7**(2), 81–4.

MacGregor, K. G., Ahmedzai, S. & Riley, J. (1994) Symptomatic relief of excoriating skin conditions using a topical thermoreversible gel. *Palliative Medicine*, **8**(1), 76–7.

Mahon, S. M. (1987) Nursing interventions for the patient with a myocutaneous flap. *Cancer Nursing*, **10**(1), 21–31.

Mahony, C. (1999) Aids to help district nurses boost patient nutrition and wound care. *Nursing Times*, **95**(32), 49–51.

Maksud, D. P. (1992) Nursing management of patients following combined free flap mandible reconstruction. *Plastic Surgical Nursing*, **12**(3), 95–105.

Mallett, J. (1997) *Nurse–Patient Haemodialysis Sessions: Orchestrated Institutional Communication and Mundane Conversations.* Ph.D. Thesis, Open University.

Mallett, J. & Dougherty, L. (2000) *The Royal Marsden Hospital Manual of Clinical Nursing Procedures*, 5th edn. Blackwell Science, Oxford.

Mallett, J., Faithfull, S., Guerrero, D. & Rhys-Evans, F. (1997) Nurse prescribing by protocol. *Nursing Times*, **93**(8), 50–52.

Mallett, J., McElligot, L., Lake, B. & Root, T. (1998) *Recommendations for the Assessment of Competency to Administer or Supply Medicines Under Group Protocols. Implications of the 'Crown Report'.* Paper presented to Patient Services Committee October meeting. Available from The Royal Marsden Hospital, London.

Mallett, J., Mulholland, J., Laverty, D., Fuller, F., Baxter, A., Faithfull, S. & Fenlon, D. (1999) An integrated approach to wound management. *International Journal of Palliative Nursing*, **5**(3), 124–32.

Martin, E. A. (ed.) (1996) *Concise Colour Medical Dictionary.* Oxford University Press.

Martin, S. J., Corrado, O. J. & Kay, E. A. (1996) Enzymatic debridement for necrotic wounds. *Journal of Wound Care*, **5**(7), 310–11.

MCA (2000) *Sale, Supply and Administration of Medicines by Health Professionals Under Patient Group Directions.* Consultation letter (MLX260) and accompanying draft guidance, (Online), Medicines Control Agency, available from URL: http://www.open.gov.uk/mca/mcahome.htm, (accessed 24 July 2000).

McCain, D. & Sutherland, S. (1998) Nursing essentials: skin grafts for patients with burns. *American Journal of Nursing*, **98**(7), 34–8.

McConn, R. (1987) Skin changes following bone marrow transplantation. *Cancer Nursing*, **10**(2), 82–4.

References

McGregor, I. A. (1989) *Fundamental Techniques of Plastic Surgery and their Surgical Applications*, 8th Edn. Churchill Livingstone, Edinburgh.

Meadows, C. (1997) Stoma and fistula care. In: *Nursing in Gastroenterology* (eds L. Bruce & T. M. D. Finlay), pp. 85–118, Churchill Livingstone, Edinburgh.

Mendez-Eastman, S. (1998) When wounds won't heal. *RN*, **61**(6), 20–23.

Middleton, K. (1990) Sugar pastes in wound management, *Dressings Times*, (Online), **3**(2), available from URL: http://www.smtl.co.uk/WMPRC/DressingsTimes/vol3.2.txt (Accessed 27 June 2000).

Miller, M. (1996) The principles of optimum wound management. *Nursing Standard*, **10**(43), 47–52.

Miller, M. (1998a) Moist wound healing: the evidence. *Nursing Times*, **94**(45), 74–6.

Miller, M. (1998b) How do I diagnose and treat wound infection? *British Journal of Nursing*, **7**(6), 335–8.

Miller, M. (1999) Nursing assessment of patients with non-acute wounds. *British Journal of Nursing*, **8**(1), 10–16.

Miller, M. & Dyson, M. (1996) *Principles of Wound Care*. Macmillan Magazines Ltd, London.

Milward, P. A. (1995) Common problems associated with necrotic and sloughy wounds. *British Journal of Nursing*, **4**(15), 896–900.

Molan, P. C. (1999a) The role of honey in the management of wounds. *Journal of Wound Care*, **8**(8), 415–18.

Molan, P. C. (1999b) *The Role of Honey in Wound Care*, (Online) Honey New Zealand. available from: http://www.honeynz.co.nz/publicat.htm (accessed 23 June 2000).

Molan, P. C. (1999c) *Why Honey is Effective as a Medicine*, (Online) Honey New Zealand, available from: http://www.honeynz.co.nz/publicat1.htm (accessed 23 June 2000).

Molan, P. C. (1999d) *A Brief Review of the Clinical Literature on the Use of Honey as a Wound Dressing*, (Online) Honey New Zealand, available from: http://www.honeynz.co.nz/publicat3.htm (accessed 23 June 2000).

Moody, M. & Grocott, P. (1993) Let use extend our knowledge base: assessment and management of fungating malignant wounds. *Professional Nurse*, June, 586–90.

Moore, D. J. (1996) The use of antiseptics in wound care, critique III. *Journal of Wound Care*, **5**(1), 46–7.

Moore, P. & Foster, L. (1998a) Acute surgical wound care 1: an overview of treatment. *British Journal of Nursing*, **7**(18), 1101–106.

Moore, P. & Foster, L. (1998b) Acute surgical wound care 2: The wound healing process. *British Journal of Nursing*, **7**(19), 1183–7.

Moore, Z. (1997a) Continuing education module 2: wound care part 5: holistic patient assessment in wound care. *The World of Irish Nursing*, **5**(5), 15–16.

Moore, Z. (1997b) Continuing education module 2: wound care part 6: local wound assessment. *The World of Irish Nursing*, **5**(6), 15–16.

Morgan, D. A. (1997) *Formulary of Wound Management Products*, 7th edn (revised). Euromed Communications Ltd, Haslemere, UK.

Morison, M. J. (1992) *A Colour Guide to the Nursing Management of Wounds*. Wolfe Publishing Ltd, London.

Mortimer, P. S. (1998) Management of skin problems medical aspects. In: *Oxford Textbook of Palliative Medicine*, 2nd edn (eds D. Doyle, G. W. C. Hanks & N. MacDonald), pp. 617–27. Oxford University Press.

Morykwas, M. J. & Argenta, L. C. (1997) Nonsurgical modalities to enhance healing and care of soft tissue wounds. *Journal of the Southern Orthopaedic Association*, **6**(4), 279–88.

Morykwas, M. J., Argenta, L. C., Shelton-Brown, E. I. & McGuirt, W. (1997) Vacuum-assisted closure: a new method for wound control and treatment: animal studies and basic foundation. *Annals of Plastic Surgery*, **38**(6), 553–62.

Munro, K. J. G. (1995) Treatment of hypertrophic and keloid scars. *Journal of Wound Care*, **4**(5), 243–5.

Murphy, A. (1995) Cleansing solution. *Nursing Times*, **91**(30), 79.

Naylor, W. (2000) *Development of a Symptom Self-Assessment Tool for Patients with Malignant Cutaneous Wounds*. BSc(Hons) Dissertation, University of Manchester.

Newman, V., Allwood, M. & Oakes, R. A. (1989) The use of metronidazole gel to control the smell of malodorous lesions. *Palliative Medicine*, **34**, 303–305.

Newton, H. & Hutchings, P. (1999) *Re-visiting Traditional Wound Care: The Use of Sugar Paste to Promote Healing*. Poster presentation at the 9th European Conference on Advances in Wound Management.

Olde Damink, S. W. M. & Soeters, P. B. (1997) Nutrition and wound healing. *Nursing Times*, **93**(30), insert 1–6.

Oliver, L. (1997) Wound cleansing. *Nursing Standard*, **11**(20), 47–51.

Parker, G. & Rendell, E. (1994) Hungry Healers. *Nursing Times*, **90**(24), 55–8.

Peate, I. & Lancaster, J. (2000) Safe use of medical gases in the clinical setting: practical tips. *British Journal of Nursing*, **9**(4), 231–6.

Peel, K. (1993) Making sense of leeches. *Nursing Times*, **89**(27), 34–5.

Pennery, E., Speechley, V. & Carroll, S. (2000) Care in context: assessment, communication and consent. In: *The Royal Marsden Hospital Manual of Clinical Nursing Procedures*, 5th edn (eds J. Mallett & L. Dougherty), pp. 1–32. Blackwell Science, Oxford.

PHLS (1999) *Surgical Site Infection. Analysis of a Year's Surveillance in English Hospitals 1997–1998*. Public Health Laboratory Service, London.

Pickworth, J. J. & De Sousa, N. (1988) Differential wound angiogenesis: quantitation by immunohistological staining for factor VIII-related antigen. In: *Beyond Occlusion:*

Wound Care Proceedings Royal Society of Medicine International Congress and Symposium Series, No. 136, (ed. T. J. Ryan), pp. 19–24. Royal Society of Medicine, London.

Pilsworth, T., Pye, D. & Roberts, A. (1995) Symptom control in advanced cancer. In: *Cancer Care: Prevention, Treatment and Palliation*, (ed. J. Davic), pp. 262–303, Chapman & Hall, London.

Porock, D., Kristjanson, L., Nikoletti, S., Cameron, F. & Pedler, P. (1998) Predicting the severity of radiation skin reactions in women with breast cancer. *Oncology Nursing Forum*, **25**(6), 1019–29.

Postmes, T., van den Bogaard, A. E. & Hazen, M. (1993) Honey for wounds, ulcers, and skin graft preservation. *The Lancet*, **341**, 756–7.

Poston, J. (1996) Sharp debridement of devitalised tissue: the nurse's role. *British Journal of Nursing*, **5**(11), 655–62.

Poteete, V. (1993) Case study: eliminating odours from wounds. *Decubitus*, **6**(4), 43–6.

Rang, H. (1995) *Pharmacology*, 3rd edn. Churchill Livingstone, Edinburgh.

Rice, A. M. (1997) An introduction to radiotherapy. *Nursing Standard*, **12**(3), 49–56.

Rigter, B., Clendon, H. & Kettle, S. (1994) Skin reactions due to radiotherapy. *New Zealand Practice Nurse*, September, 17–22.

Robinson, B. J. (2000) The use of a hydrofibre dressings in wound management. *Journal of Wound Care*, **9**(1), 32–4.

Rodeheaver, G. T. (1999) Pressure ulcer debridement and cleansing: a review of current literature. *Ostomy/Wound Management*, **45**(1A) Suppl.

Rodzwic, D. & Donnard, J. (1986) The use of myocutaneous flaps in reconstructive surgery for head and neck cancer: guidelines for nursing care. *Oncology Nursing Forum*, **13**(3), 29–34.

Rolstad, B. S., Borchert, K., Magnan, S. & Scheel, N. (1994) A comparison of an alcohol-based and siloxane-based peri-wound skin protectant. *Journal of Wound Care*, **3**(8), 367–8.

Ross, M. H., Romrell, L. J. & Kaye, G. I. (1995) *Histology A Text and Atlas*, 3rd edn. Williams and Wilkins, Baltimore, Maryland, USA.

Rutter, P. M., Carpenter, B., Hill S. S. & Locke I. C. (2000) Varidase: the science behind the medicament. *Journal of Wound Care*, **9**(5), 223–6.

Saunders, J. & Regnard, C. (1989) Management of malignant ulcers – a flow diagram. *Palliative Medicine*, **3**, 153–5.

Schneider, A. M., Morykwas, M. J. & Argenta, L. C. (1998) A new and reliable method of securing skin grafts to difficult recipient bed. *Journal of Plastic and Reconstructive Surgery*, **102**(4), 1195–8.

Schulte, M. (1993) Yoghurt helps to control wound odour. *Oncology Nursing Forum*, **20**(8), 1262.

Sherman, R. A. (1996) *Maggot Therapy Project*, (Online), available from URL: http://www.ucihs.uci.edu/path/sherman/home pg.htm (accessed 23 June 2000).

Sherman, R. (1998) Maggot debridement in modern medicine. *Infectious Medicine*, **15**(9), 651–6.

Silver, I. A. (1994) The physiology of wound healing. *Journal of Wound Care*, **3**(2), 106–109.

Sitton, E. (1992) Early and late radiation-induced skin alterations part 1: mechanisms of skin changes. *Oncology Nursing Forum*, **19**(5), 801–807.

Sleigh, J. W. & Linter, S. P. K. (1985) Lesson of the week: hazards of hydrogen peroxide. *British Medical Journal*, **291**, 1706.

SMTL (1995) *A Prescriber's Guide to Dressings and Wound Management Materials*, (Online). Surgical Materials Testing Laboratory, Bridgend General Hospital, Mid Glamorgan, available from URL: http://www.smtl.co.uk/WMPRC/VFM-report/OLD/allguide.html (accessed 27 September 1999).

SMTL (1999) *Dressing Data Cards*, (Online). Available from URL: http://www.smtl.co.uk/WMPRC/DataCards/html (accessed 24 August 1999).

Souhami, R. & Tobias, J. (1998) *Cancer and its Management*. Blackwell Science, Oxford.

Southwest Technologies Inc (2000) *Elasto-Gel Wound Care*, (Online), available from URL: http://www.elastogel.com/Elasto-Gel.htm (accessed 27 July 2000).

Sparrow, G., Minton, M., Rubens, R. D., Simmons, N. A. & Aubrey, C. (1980) Metronidazole in smelly tumours. *Lancet*, **1**(8179), 1185.

Stein, C. (1995) The control of pain in peripheral tissue by opioids. *The New England Journal of Medicine*, **332**(25), 1685–90.

Sterling, C. (1996) Methods of wound assessment documentation: a study. *Nursing Standard*, **11**(10), 38–41.

Stevens, J. (1998) Hydrogels and foams in combination. *Journal of Wound Care*, **7**(5), 235.

Stocum, D. L. (1995) *Molecular Biology Intelligence Unit. Wound Repair, Regeneration and Artificial Tissues*. R.G. Landes Company, Austin, Texas.

Strete, D. (1995) *A Color Atlas of Histology*. HarperCollins College Publishers, New York.

Subrahmanyam, M. (1991) Topical application of honey in treatment of burns. *British Journal of Surgery*, **78**(4), 497–8.

Sussman, C. (1998) Wound healing biology and chronic wound healing. In: *Wound Care, A Collaborative Practice Manual for Physical Therapists and Nurses* (eds

C. Sussman & B. M. Bate-Jensen), pp. 31–47. Aspen Publishers, Gaithersberg, Maryland, USA.

Tatnall, F. M., Leigh, I. M. & Gibson, J. R. (1990) Comparative study of antiseptic toxicity on basal keratinocytes and fibroblasts. *Skin Pharmacology*, **3**(3), 157–63.

Thomas, A. M. L., Harding, K. G. & Moore, K. (1999) The structure and composition of chronic wound eschar. *Journal of Wound Care*, **8**(6), 285–7.

Thomas Hess, C. (1998) *Nurse's Clinical Guide. Wound Care*, 2nd edn. Springhouse Corporation, Pennsylvania.

Thomas, S. (1990) *Wound Management and Dressings*. Pharmaceutical Press, London.

Thomas, S. (1992a) *Current Practices in the Management of Fungating Lesions and Radiation Damaged Skin*. The Surgical Materials Testing Laboratory, Bridgend Hospital, Mid Glamorgan.

Thomas, S. (1992b) Alginates; a guide to the properties and uses of the different alginate dressings available today. *Journal of Wound Care*, **1**(1), 29–32.

Thomas, S. (1994) *Handbook of Wound Dressings 1994 Edition*. Macmillan Magazines Ltd, London.

Thomas, S. (1997) A structured approach to the selection of dressings. *World Wide Wounds*, (Online), available from URL: http://www.smtl.co.uk/World-Wide-Wounds/1997/july/Thomas-Guide/Dress-Select.html (accessed 19 October 1999).

Thomas, S. (1998) The importance of secondary dressings in wound care. *Journal of Wound Care*, **7**(4), 189–92.

Thomas, S. & Jones, M. (1999) *The Use of Sterile Maggots in Wound Care*. Educational Leaflet, **6**(4). The Wound Care Society, Huntingdon, UK.

Thomas, S., Andrews, A. & Jones, M. (1998a) The use of larval therapy in wound management. *Journal of Wound Care*, **7**(10), 521–4.

Thomas, S., Fisher, B., Fram, P. & Waring, M. (1998b) Odour absorbing dressings: a comparative laboratory study. *World Wide Wounds*, (Online), available from URL: http://www.smtl.co.uk/World-Wide-Wounds/1998/march/Odour-Absorbing-Dressings/odour-absorbing-dressings.html (accessed 28 June 2000).

Thomas, S., Vowden, K. & Newton, H. (1998c) Combining hydrogel and foam dressings. *Journal of Wound Care*, **7**(3), 154.

Thomas, S., Andrews, A., Hay, P. & Bourgoise, S. (1999a) The anti-microbial activity of maggot secretions: results of a preliminary study. *Journal of Tissue Viability*, **9**(6), 127–32.

Thomas, S., Jones, M., Shutler, S. & Jones, S. (1999b) *Maggots in Wound Debridement – an Introduction*, (Online). Surgical Materials Testing Laboratory, Bridgend, available from URL: http://www.smtl.co.uk/WMPRC/Maggots/maggots.html (accessed 23 June 2000).

Thomas, S. (2000) Alginate dressings in surgery and wound management – part 1. *Journal of Wound Care*, **9**(2), 56–60.

Thomson, P. (1998) The microbiology of wounds. *Journal of Wound Care*, **7**(9), 477–8.

Iopham, J. (1991) Experiences with sugar paste in zanzibar. *Dressings Times*, (Online), **4**(3), available from URL: http://www.smtl.co.uk/WMPRC/ DressingsTimes/vol4.3.txt (accessed 28 June 2000).

Tortora, G. J. & Grabowski, S. R. (1996) *Principles of Anatomy and Physiology*, 8th edn. Harper Collins, Menlo Park, Ca.

Trevelyn, J. (1996) Wound cleansing: principles and practice. *Nursing Times*, **92**(16), 46–8.

UKCC (1992) *The Scope of Professional Practice*. United Kingdom Central Council for Nursing, Midwifery and Health Visiting, London.

UKCC (1998) *Guidelines for Records and Record Keeping*. United Kingdom Central Council for Nursing, Midwifery and Health Visiting, London.

Van Toller, S. (1994) Invisible wounds: the effects of skin ulcer malodours. *Journal of Wound Care*, **3**(2), 103–105.

Voge, C. & Lehnherr, S. M. (1999) Get attached to leeches. *Nursing*, **29**(11), 46–7.

Vowden, K. (1995) Common problems in wound care: wound and ulcer measurement. *British Journal of Nursing*, **4**(13), 775–9.

Vowden, K. R. & Vowden, P. (1999a) Wound debridement, part 1: non-sharp techniques. *Journal of Wound Care*, **8**(5), 237–40.

Vowden, K. R. & Vowden, P. (1999b) Wound debridement, part 2: sharp techniques. *Journal of Wound Care*, **8**(6), 291–4.

Weinberg, R. A. (1996) How cancer arises. *Scientific America*, **275**(3), 62–70.

Wells, L. (1994) At the front line of care, the importance of nutrition in wound management. *Professional Nurse*, May, 525–30.

Wells, M., Manktelow, R., Boyd, V. & Bowen, J. (1993) *The Medical Leech: An Old Treatment Revisited*. Wiley-Liss Inc, Toronto.

Werner, K. G. (1999) *Guideline for the Outpatient Treatment of Pressure Ulcer*, (Online). Compliance Network Physicians/Health Force Initiative, Inc, available from URL: http://www.cnhfi.org/pressure-ulcer.html (accessed 8 October 1999).

Westlake, C. (1991) Commitment to function: microsurgical flaps. *Plastic Surgical Nursing*, **11**(3), 95–100.

Westmore, M. G. (1991) Make-up as an adjunct and aid to the practice of dermatology. *Dermatologic Clinics*, **9**(1), 81–8.

References

WHRU (1996) *Honey as an Antimicrobial Agent*, (Online). Waikato Honey Research Unit, University of Waikato, New Zealand, available from: http://honey.bio.waikato.ac.nz/honey intro.shtml (accessed 3 July 2000).

Wilkinson, B. (1997) Hard Graft. *Nursing Times*, **93**(16), 63–8.

Williams, C. (1994) Product focus Sorbsan®. *British Journal of Nursing*, **3**(13), 677–80.

Williams, C. (1995a) Product focus Allevyn®. *British Journal of Nursing*, **4**(2), 107–10.

Williams, C. (1995b) Product focus Cavi-care®. *British Journal of Nursing*, **4**(9), 526–8.

Williams, C. (1996a) Product focus Granugel®: hydrocolloid gel. *British Journal of Nursing*, **5**(3), 188–90.

Williams, C. (1996b) Product focus Cica-care®: adhesive gel sheet. *British Journal of Nursing*, **5**(14), 875–6.

Williams, C. (1998) 3M Cavilon® no sting barrier film in the protection of vulnerable skin. *British Journal of Nursing*, **7**(10), 613–15.

Williams, C. (1999a) Product focus: an investigation of the benefits of aquacel hydrofibre wound dressing. *British Journal of Nursing*, **8**(10), 676–80.

Williams, C. (1999b) Product focus: the benefits and application of the lyofoam product range. *British Journal of Nursing*, **8**(11), 745–9.

Williams, C. (1999c) Superskin: a polymer adhesive skin sealant. *Nursing and Residential Care*, **1**(1), 56–7.

Williams, C. & Young, T. (1998) *Myth and Reality in Wound Care*. Mark Allen Publishing Ltd, Dinton, Wiltshire, UK.

Wilson, J. (1995) *Infection Control in Clinical Practice*. Baillière Tindall, London.

Winter, G. A. (1962) Formation of the scab and rate of epithelialisation in the skin of the young domestic pig. *Nature*, **193**, 293–5.

Young, T. (1997) Wound care: the challenge of managing fungating wounds. *Community Nurse* **3**(9), 41–4.

Young, T. (1998) Reaping the benefits of foam dressings. *Community Nurse*, **4**(5), 47–8.

Young, T. & Fowler, A. (1998) Nursing management of skin grafts and donor sites. *British Journal of Nursing*, **7**(6), 324–34.

Further Reading

Carney, S. (1993) Hypertrophic scar formation after skin surgery. *Journal of Wound Care*, **2**(5), 299–302.

Collier, M. (1997) The assessment of patients with malignant fungating wounds – a holistic approach: part 2. *Nursing Times*, **93**(46), Suppl. 1–4.

Cooper, R., Bale, S. & Harding, K. G. (1995) An improved cleansing regime for a modified foam cavity dressing. *Journal of Wound Care*, **4**(1), 13–16.

Fairbairn, K. (1994) A challenge that requires further research: management of fungating breast lesions. *Professional Nurse*, January, 272–7.

Gallagher, J. (1995) Management of cutaneous symptoms. *Seminars in Oncology Nursing*, **11**(4), 239–47.

Grocott, P. (1999) The management of fungating wounds. *Journal of Wound Care*, **8**(5), 232–4.

Heenan, A. (1998) Dressings on the drug tariff. *World Wide Wounds* (Online), available from URL: http://www.smtl.co.uk/World-Wide-Wounds/1997/july/Heenan/Tariff.html (accessed 27 October 1999).

Johnson, A. (1987) Wound care: packing cavities. *Nursing Times*, **83**(36), 59–62.

Leaper, D. (1988) Antiseptic toxicity in open wounds. *Nursing Times*, **84**(25), 77–9.

Manning, M. P. (1998) Metastasis to skin. *Seminars in Oncology Nursing*, **14**(3), 240–43.

Margolin, S. G., Breneman, J. C., Denman, D. L., LaChapelle, P., Weckbach, L. & Aron, B. S. (1990) Management of radiation-induced moist skin desquamation using hydrocolloid dressing. *Cancer Nursing*, **13**(2), 71–80.

McGregor, F. & Baxter, H. (1999) Staying power. *Nursing Times*, **95**(19), 66–71.

Price, E. (1996) The stigma of smell. *Nursing Times*, **92**(20), 70–72.

Pudner, R. (1998) The management of patients with a fungating or malignant wound. *Journal of Community Nursing*, (Online), **12**(9), available from URL: http://www.jcn.co.uk/septfung.htm (accessed 18 February 2000).

Ryan, T. J. (1985) *An Environment for Healing: The Role of Occlusion. International Congress and Symposium Series*, No. 88. The Royal Society of Medicine, London.

Yancey, R., Given, B. A., White, N. J., DeVoss, D. & Coyle, B. (1998) Computerized documentation for a rural nursing interventions project. *Computer Nursing*, **16**(5), 275–84.

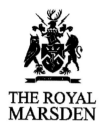

THE ROYAL MARSDEN

Appendix

Patient Group Direction for the
Management of Fungating Wounds:
Supply and Administration of
Wound Management Products

PLAN OF CARE

Diagnosis/condition	Fungating/complex wound
(Potential) symptom(s)/clinical criteria under which the patient will be eligible for inclusion in the protocol	Fungating/complex wound Difficulty with controlling/containing symptoms associated with wound
Aims of treatment or care	Minimise symptoms and improve patient comfort
Criteria under which the patient will be excluded from care within the protocol	Initial assessment indicates a wound that is due to vascular disease that may require surgical assessment
Actions to be taken for patients who are excluded from treatment under the protocol	Referral to physician/surgeon
Actions to be taken for patients who do not wish to receive, or do not adhere to, care under the protocol	Referral to physician/surgeon for opinion Discuss reasons with patient and ensure they have adequate information to make an informed decision Care taken over by community team if being discharged home
Methods	Educate the patient and family on the rationale for the choice of wound care products Inform patient of potential problems with wound care products Ensure the patient and family understand the information given Ascertain who may be dressing the wound at home (may be the family/patient/carer), so that they receive adequate information regarding methods of wound management
Identification and management of adverse reactions	Hypersensitivity/allergy (e.g. erythema, inflammation) to wound care product may occur. In this instance stop use of product and select an alternative with input from a pharmacist If increased breakdown of the wound and/or surrounding skin occurs, remove the dressing product immediately and inform medical staff

Continued

	If exacerbation of existing symptoms occurs (e.g. increased exudate, odour or pain) check for other possible reasons, such as infection, and treat. If necessary select an alternative dressing product
Follow-up treatment which may be required	Monitor treatment and care as appropriate (e.g. via telephone consultation with community staff and at each outpatient appointment). If there are problems with the chosen wound management products, advise the community staff, patient and carer of alternative products in liaison with the patient's GP.
Evaluation of treatment/care (see also audit trail)	Assess, or ask the patient to assess, any changes in, and the management of, wound related symptoms. Evaluate the efficacy of dressings via community staff and/or during outpatient appointments. Evaluate and document care. Complete audit trail to enable care for the patient group to be assessed

MEDICINE*

Medicine	Alginates (e.g. Sorbsan®)
Legal status of medicine	Medical device
Mode of action	To accelerate healing process To deslough a wound To contain exudate
Indications for treatment	To contain symptoms (moderate to heavy exudate, slough) To aid wound healing, if appropriate To provide comfort
Concurrent medicines	None to check as there is no systemic uptake (BNF 2000).
Dose range within which medicine can be supplied or	A combination of dressings used in conjunction with the wound management guidelines

*Medicine and/or medical advice.

Continued

administered	(Laverty *et al.* 2000b) related to symptom management. Dressing changes should range from once a day to once every 3–4 days depending on symptom control and changing needs
Criteria for deciding dose and changes in dose within above range	Symptom changes related to changing circumstances, e.g. infection To provide comfort
Frequency of administration and maximum number of doses if more than one dose required	Range from daily to once every 3–4 days
Period of time over which the medicine can be administered	As long as the wound is evident/causing problems
Method or route of administration of medicine	Topical to wound
Indications for review	Regular assessment as appropriate by telephone contact to community nursing teams and/or with the patient/carer in the outpatient setting Refer to evaluation of treatment section
Rationale for referral to physicians and arrangements for achieving this	Referral to physician if hypersensitivity/allergic reaction occurs Referral to surgeon if wound is post-operative
Incompatible medicines	None stated in data sheets
Contra-indications, interactions and side effects	Known hypersensitivity and/or allergy to product (data source: patient information sheets from manufacturer)
Reporting of suspected adverse drug reactions	These should be reported immediately to relevant doctor and pharmacist and documented in patient's clinical notes
Arrangements for pharmacovigilance communications and amendments to protocols as the result of new safety information	This will be carried out by the doctor or pharmacist and will minimally include reporting of adverse incidents, communication of new safety information, withdrawal of drugs etc. between relevant professionals and also to external agencies. This should be documented and reported to the Medical Devices Agency

MEDICINE

Medicine	Barrier films (e.g. Cavilon®)
Legal status of medicine	Medical device
Mode of action	To accelerate healing process To protect the skin To prevent infection
Indications for treatment	To contain symptoms (skin excoriation/maceration, tape stripping) To aid wound healing, if appropriate To provide comfort To prevent skin breakdown
Concurrent medicines	None to check as there is no systemic uptake
Dose range within which medicine can be supplied or administered	A combination of dressings used in conjunction with the wound management guidelines (Laverty *et al.* 2000b) related to symptom management. Dressing changes should range from once a day to once every 3 days depending on symptom control and changing needs
Criteria for deciding dose and changes in dose within above range	Symptom changes related to changing circumstances, e.g. infection To provide comfort
Frequency of administration and maximum number of doses if more than one dose required	Range from daily to every 72 hours
Period of time over which the medicine can be administered	As long as the wound is evident/demonstrating identified problems
Method or route of administration of medicine	Topical to skin
Indications for review	Regular assessment as appropriate by telephone contact to community nursing teams and/or with the patient/carer in the outpatient setting Refer to evaluation of treatment section

Continued

Rationale for referral to physicians and arrangements for achieving this	Referral to physician if hypersensitivity/allergic reaction occurs Referral to surgeon if wound is postoperative
Incompatible medicines	None stated in data sheets
Contra-indications, Interactions and side effects	Known hypersensitivity and/or allergy to product (data source: patient information sheets from manufacturer)
Reporting of suspected adverse drug reactions	These should be reported immediately to relevant doctor and pharmacist and documented in patient's clinical notes
Arrangements for pharmacovigilance communications and amendments to protocols as the result of new safety information	This will be carried out by the doctor or pharmacist and will minimally include reporting of adverse incidents, communication of new safety information, withdrawal of drugs etc. between relevant professionals and also to external agencies. This should be documented and reported to the Medical Devices Agency

MEDICINE

Medicine	Debriding enzymes (e.g. Varidase®)
Legal status of medicine	POM
Mode of action	To accelerate healing process To deslough/break down necrotic tissue To prevent infection
Indications for treatment	To contain symptoms (eschar, slough, infection) To aid wound healing, if appropriate
Concurrent medicines	Intravenous streptokinase (avoid use within 6 months of topical application of Varidase®) (Morgan 1997)
Dose range within which medicine can be supplied or administered	A combination of dressings used in conjunction with the wound management guidelines (Laverty et al. 2000b) related to symptom management. Dressing changes should range from once to twice a day depending on symptom control and changing needs

Continued

Criteria for deciding dose and changes in dose within above range	Symptom changes related to changing circumstances, e.g. infection To provide comfort
Frequency of administration and maximum number of doses if more than one dose required	Range once to twice daily
Period of time over which the medicine can be administered	As long as the wound is evident/demonstrating identified problems
Method or route of administration of medicine	Topical to wound
Indications for review	Regular assessment as appropriate by telephone contact to community nursing teams and/or with the patient/carer in the outpatient setting Refer to evaluation of treatment section
Rationale for referral to physicians and arrangements for achieving this	Referral to physician if hypersensitivity/allergic reaction occurs Referral to surgeon if wound is postoperative
Incompatible medicines	Intravenous streptokinase
Contra-indications, interactions and side effects	Known hypersensitivity and/or allergy to product Active bleeding from the wound Patients at risk of myocardial infarction Allergic reaction (infrequent) Transient burning sensation (Data source: Morgan 1997, BNF 2000)
Reporting of suspected adverse drug reactions	These should be reported immediately to relevant doctor and pharmacist and documented in patient's clinical notes
Arrangements for pharmacovigilance communications and amendments to protocols as the result of new safety information	This will be carried out by the doctor or pharmacist and will minimally include reporting of adverse incidents, communication of new safety information, withdrawal of drugs etc. between relevant professionals and also to external agencies. This should be documented in the Report on Suspected Adverse Drug Reactions (BNF 2000) sheet and should be completed by doctor and pharmacist

MEDICINE

Medicine	Foams (to include hydrosorbtive dressings) (e.g. Allevyn® Hydrocellular, Allevyn® Cavity, CombiDerm® (N))
Legal status of medicine	Medical device
Mode of action	To accelerate healing process To contain waste products from wound breakdown To prevent infection
Indications for treatment	To contain symptoms (moderate to high exudate) To aid wound healing, if appropriate To provide comfort
Concurrent medicines	None to check as there is no systemic uptake (BNF 2000)
Dose range within which medicine can be supplied or administered	A combination of dressings used in conjunction with the wound management guidelines (Laverty *et al.* 2000b) related to symptom management. Dressing changes should range from once or twice a day to once every 7 days depending on symptom control and changing needs
Criteria for deciding dose and changes in dose within above range	Symptom changes related to changing circumstances, e.g. infection To provide comfort
Frequency of administration and maximum number of doses if more than one dose required	Range from twice daily to once every 7 days
Period of time over which the medicine can be administered	As long as the wound is evident/demonstrating identified problems
Method or route of administration of medicine	Topical to wound
Indications for review	Regular assessment as appropriate by telephone contact to community nursing teams and/or with the patient/carer in the outpatient setting Refer to evaluation of treatment section

Continued

Rationale for referral to physicians and arrangements for achieving this	Referral to physician if hypersensitivity/allergic reaction occurs Referral to surgeon if wound is post-operative
Incompatible medicines	None stated in data sheets
Contra-indications, interactions and side effects	Known hypersensitivity and/or allergy to product (data source: patient information sheets from manufacturer)
Reporting of suspected adverse drug reactions	These should be reported immediately to relevant doctor and pharmacist and documented in patient's clinical notes
Arrangements for pharmacovigilance communications and amendments to protocols as the result of new safety information	This will be carried out by the doctor or pharmacist and will minimally include reporting of adverse incidents, communication of new safety information, withdrawal of drugs etc. between relevant professionals and also to external agencies. This should be documented and reported to the Medical Devices Agency

MEDICINE

Medicine	Hydrocolloid (e.g. Granuflex®, Duoderm E®)
Legal status of medicine	Medical device
Mode of action	To accelerate healing process To deslough a wound To prevent infection To contain low to moderate exudate
Indications for treatment	To contain symptoms (light to moderate exudate, slough, odour) To aid wound healing, if appropriate To provide comfort
Concurrent medicines	None to check as there is no systemic uptake (BNF 2000)

Continued

Dose range within which medicine can be supplied or administered	A combination of dressings used in conjunction with the wound management guidelines (Laverty *et al.* 2000b) related to symptom management. Dressing changes should range from once or twice a day to once every 7 days depending on symptom control and changing needs
Criteria for deciding dose and changes in dose within above range	Symptom changes related to changing circumstances, e.g. infection To provide comfort
Frequency of administration and maximum number of doses if more than one dose required	Range from daily to once every 7 days
Period of time over which the medicine can be administered	As long as the wound is evident/demonstrating identified problems
Method or route of administration of medicine	Topical to wound
Indications for review	Regular assessment as appropriate by telephone contact to community nursing teams and/or with the patient/carer in the outpatient setting Refer to evaluation of treatment section
Rationale for referral to physicians and arrangements for achieving this	Referral to physician if hypersensitivity/allergic reaction occurs Referral to surgeon if wound is postoperative
Incompatible medicines	None stated in data sheets
Contra-indications, interactions and side effects	Known hypersensitivity and/or allergy to product Heavy exudate (data source: patient information sheets from manufacturer)
Reporting of suspected adverse drug reactions	These should be reported immediately to relevant doctor and pharmacist and documented in patient's clinical notes
Arrangements for pharmacovigilance communications and amendments to protocols as the result of new safety information	This will be carried out by the doctor or pharmacist and will minimally include reporting of adverse incidents, communication of new safety information, withdrawal of drugs etc. between relevant professionals and also to external agencies. This should be documented and reported to the Medical Devices Agency

MEDICINE

Medicine	Hydrofibre (e.g. Aquacel®)
Legal status of medicine	Medical Device
Mode of action	To accelerate healing process To absorb medium to high amounts of exudate To deslough a wound To prevent infection
Indications for treatment	To contain symptoms (medium to high exudate, slough) To aid wound healing, if appropriate To provide comfort
Concurrent medicines	None to check as there is no systemic uptake (BNF 2000)
Dose range within which medicine can be supplied or administered	A combination of dressings used in conjunction with the wound management guidelines (Laverty et al. 2000b) related to symptom management. Dressing changes should range from once or twice a day to once every 7 days depending on symptom control and changing needs
Criteria for deciding dose and changes in dose within above range	Symptom changes related to changing circumstances, e.g. infection To provide comfort
Frequency of administration and maximum number of doses if more than one dose required	Range from twice daily to once every 7 days
Period of time over which the medicine can be administered	As long as the wound is evident/demonstrating identified problems
Method or route of administration of medicine	Topical to wound
Indications for review	Regular assessment as appropriate by telephone contact to community nursing teams and/or with the patient/carer in the outpatient setting Refer to evaluation of treatment section
Rationale for referral to physicians and arrangements for achieving this	Referral to physician if hypersensitivity/allergic reaction occurs Referral to surgeon if wound is postoperative

Continued

Incompatible medicines	None stated in data sheets
Contra-indications, interactions and side effects	Known hypersensitivity and/or allergy to product Dry, necrotic wounds (data source: patient information sheets from manufacturer)
Reporting of suspected adverse drug reactions	These should be reported immediately to relevant doctor and pharmacist and documented in patient's clinical notes
Arrangements for pharmacovigilance communications and amendments to protocols as the result of new safety information	This will be carried out by the doctor or pharmacist and will minimally include reporting of adverse incidents, communication of new safety information, withdrawal of drugs etc. between relevant professionals and also to external agencies. This should be documented and reported to the Medical Devices Agency

MEDICINE

Medicine	Hydrogel (e.g. Granugel®)
Legal status of medicine	Medical device
Mode of action	To accelerate healing process To debride slough and eschar
Indications for treatment	To contain symptoms (slough, eschar, light to moderate exudate) To aid wound healing, if appropriate To provide comfort
Concurrent medicines	None to check as there is no systemic uptake (BNF 2000)
Dose range within which medicine can be supplied or administered	A combination of dressings used in conjunction with the wound management guidelines (Laverty et al. 2000b) related to symptom management. Dressing changes should range from once or twice a day to once every 7 days depending on symptom control and changing needs
Criteria for deciding dose and changes in dose within above range	Symptom changes related to changing circumstances, e.g. infection To provide comfort

Continued

Frequency of administration and maximum number of doses if more than one dose required	Range from twice daily to once every 7 days
Period of time over which the medicine can be administered	As long as the wound is evident/demonstrating identified problems
Method or route of administration of medicine	Topical to wound
Indications for review	Regular assessment as appropriate by telephone contact to community nursing teams and/or with the patient/carer in the outpatient setting Refer to evaluation of treatment section
Rationale for referral to physicians and arrangements for achieving this	Referral to physician if hypersensitivity/allergic reaction occurs Referral to surgeon if wound is postoperative
Incompatible medicines	None stated in data sheets
Contraindications, interactions and side effects	Known hypersensitivity and/or allergy to product Anaerobic infection (data source: patient information sheets from manufacturer (Morgan 1997). Heavily exuding wounds
Reporting of suspected adverse drug reactions	These should be reported immediately to relevant doctor and pharmacist and documented in patient's clinical notes
Arrangements for pharmacovigilance communications and amendments to protocols as the result of new safety information	This will be carried out by the doctor or pharmacist and will minimally include reporting of adverse incidents, communication of new safety information, withdrawal of drugs etc. between relevant professionals and also to external agencies. This should be documented and reported to the Medical Devices Agency

MEDICINE

Medicine	Hydrogel sheet (e.g. Geliperm®, Novogel®)
Legal status of medicine	Medical device
Mode of action	To accelerate healing process To contain waste products from wound breakdown To prevent infection To provide moist environment
Indications for treatment	To contain symptoms (slough, eschar, light to moderate exudate) To aid wound healing, if appropriate To provide comfort
Concurrent medicines	None to check as there is no systemic uptake (BNF 2000)
Dose range within which medicine can be supplied or administered	A combination of dressings used in conjunction with the wound management guidelines (Laverty et al. 2000b) related to symptom management. Dressing changes should range from once or twice a day to once every 7 days depending on symptom control and changing needs
Criteria for deciding dose and changes in dose within above range	Symptom changes related to changing circumstances, e.g. infection To provide comfort
Frequency of administration and maximum number of doses if more than one dose required	Range from twice daily to once every 7 days
Period of time over which the medicine can be administered	As long as the wound is evident/demonstrating identified problems
Method or route of administration of medicine	Topical to wound
Indications for review	Regular assessment as appropriate by telephone contact to community nursing teams and/or with the patient/carer in the outpatient setting Refer to evaluation of treatment section

Continued

Rationale for referral to physicians and arrangements for achieving this	Referral to physician if hypersensitivity/allergic reaction occurs Referral to surgeon if wound is postoperative
Incompatible medicines	None stated in data sheets
Contra-indications, interactions and side effects	Known hypersensitivity and/or allergy to product Anaerobic infection (data source: patient information sheets from manufacturer (Morgan 1997) Deep narrow cavities or sinuses
Reporting of suspected adverse drug reactions	These should be reported immediately to relevant doctor and pharmacist and documented in patient's clinical notes
Arrangements for pharmacovigilance communications and amendments to protocols as the result of new safety information	This will be carried out by the doctor or pharmacist and will minimally include reporting of adverse incidents, communication of new safety information, withdrawal of drugs etc. between relevant professionals and also to external agencies. This should be documented and reported to the Medical Devices Agency

MEDICINE

Medicine	Metronidazole gel (e.g. Metrotop®)
Legal status of medicine	POM
Mode of action	To control malodour To treat infection
Indications for treatment	To contain symptoms (malodour) To provide comfort
Concurrent medicines	None to check as there is limited systemic absorption (Morgan 1997)
Dose range within which medicine can be supplied or administered	A combination of dressings used in conjunction with the wound management guidelines (Laverty et al. 2000b) related to symptom management. Dressing changes should range from once or twice a day to once every 7 days depending on symptom control and changing needs

Continued

Criteria for deciding dose and changes in dose within above range	Symptom changes related to changing circumstances, e.g. infection To provide comfort
Frequency of administration and maximum number of doses if more than one dose required	Range from once to twice a day
Period of time over which the medicine can be administered	As long as the wound is evident/demonstrating identified problems
Method or route of administration of medicine	Topical to wound
Indications for review	Regular assessment as appropriate by telephone contact to community nursing teams and/or with the patient/carer in the outpatient setting Refer to evaluation of treatment section
Rationale for referral to physicians and arrangements for achieving this	Referral to physician if hypersensitivity/allergic reaction occurs Referral to surgeon if wound is postoperative
Incompatible medicines	None stated in data sheets
Contra-indications, interactions and side effects	Known hypersensitivity and/or allergy to product Local skin irritation Avoid exposure to strong sunlight or UV light (data source: BNF 2000)
Reporting of suspected adverse drug reactions	These should be reported immediately to relevant doctor and pharmacist and documented in patient's clinical notes
Arrangements for pharmacovigilance communications and amendments to protocols as the result of new safety information	This will be carried out by the doctor or pharmacist and will minimally include reporting of adverse incidents, communication of new safety information, withdrawal of drugs etc. between relevant professionals and also to external agencies. This should be documented in the Report on Suspected Adverse Drug Reactions (BNF 2000) sheet and should be completed by doctor and pharmacist

MEDICINE

Medicine	Semi-permeable film (e.g. Tegaderm®)
Legal status of medicine	Medical device
Mode of action	To provide a moist wound environment To prevent skin breakdown and infection For securing of dressings
Indications for treatment	To contain symptoms To secure dressings To provide comfort
Concurrent medicines	None to check as there is no systemic uptake (BNF 2000)
Dose range within which medicine can be supplied or administered	A combination of dressings used in conjunction with the wound management guidelines (Laverty *et al.* 2000b) related to symptom management. Dressing changes should range from once or twice a day to once every 7 days depending on symptom control and changing needs
Criteria for deciding dose and changes in dose within above range	Symptom changes related to changing circumstances, e.g. infection To provide comfort
Frequency of administration and maximum number of doses if more than one dose required	Range from twice daily to once every 7 days
Period of time over which the medicine can be administered	As long as the wound is evident/demonstrating identified problems
Method or route of administration of medicine	Topical to wound
Indications for review	Regular assessment as appropriate by telephone contact to community nursing teams and/or with the patient/carer in the outpatient setting Refer to evaluation of treatment section
Rationale for referral to physicians and arrangements for achieving this	Referral to physician if hypersensitivity/allergic reaction occurs Referral to surgeon if wound is postoperative

Continued

Incompatible medicines	None stated in data sheets
Contra-indications, interactions and side effects	Known hypersensitivity and/or allergy to product Infection. Moderate and highly exuding wounds (data source: patient information sheets from manufacturer)
Reporting of suspected adverse drug reactions	These should be reported immediately to relevant doctor and pharmacist and documented in patient's clinical notes
Arrangements for pharmacovigilance communications and amendments to protocols as the result of new safety information	This will be carried out by the doctor or pharmacist and will minimally include reporting of adverse incidents, communication of new safety information, withdrawal of drugs etc. between relevant professionals and also to external agencies. This should be documented and reported to the Medical Devices Agency

AUDIT TRAIL (Records required for a documented audit trail)

Health care professional providing treatment
Patient identifiers
Patient (potential) symptoms
Medicine being provided
Adverse drug reactions
Evaluation of treatment/care
Clear documentation within clinical notes (to fulfill UKCC criteria (UKCC 1998))

AUTHORISATION OF PROTOCOL

Chief Nurse and Director of Quality Assurance's signature on behalf of Nursing and Rehabilitation Advisory Committee

Medical Director's signature on behalf of the Medical advisory Committee

Signature of Chief Pharmacist

Signature of Chair on behalf of Drugs and Therapeutics Committee

Signature of Chair on behalf of the Steering Group on Protocols and Prescribing by Non-Medical Staff

AUTHORISATION OF NURSE TO USE PROTOCOL

Signature of nurse
This confirms the nurse:
- understands the protocol
- has received the necessary education and
  training
- is of the opinion s/he is competent to
  implement the protocol effectively
- agrees to work within the protocol

Signature of relevant medical consultant as agreed by Divisional Nurse Director
Signature of Divisional Nurse Director
Date protocol agreed
Rationale for review   Initial assessment of protocol
Frequency of review   Six months
Date protocol to be reviewed (after which the
  protocol is no longer valid)
Clinical areas in which a copy of protocol to be kept

COMPETENCY OF NURSE

Nurse		
Designation		
Competency/qualifications	Indicators	Assessed
Level of assessment and care provided by nurse is sufficient for protocolised nurse administration of medicines (evidence provided by the nurse, their manager and job description)	Expert level of assessment and care provided assessed by nurse and manager	
Registered nurse and/or registered children's nurse	Appropriateness of qualifications to relevant clinical area assessed by nurse and manager	
UKCC registration	UKCC registration checked and assessed by manager	
Oncology certificate or equivalent, relevant other qualifications	Certification checked by manager	

Continued

195

Nurse		
Designation		
Competency/qualifications	Indicators	Assessed
One year's experience in relevant clinical area at senior level (minimally at 'F' grade)	Competency checked by manager	
Knowledge and understanding of key topics of pharmacy as evidenced by professional qualifications and self-assessment by the nurse (according to the statements within the Scope of Professional Practice (UKCC 1992) of general pharmacology and other relevant details of the product(s)/drug(s) concerned including:	Knowledge and understanding of key topics of pharmacy assessed by agreed Hospital assessor and nurse	

- the names of the drugs/medicines/ products concerned
- the legal status of drugs/medicines /products concerned (e.g. POM, P, GSL or Medical Device)
- dose and/or permissible dose range and the criteria for deciding on the dose to be administered or recommended
- method and route of administration
- if more than one dose is required, the permitted frequency of administration
- the permitted total dose and maximum number of doses allowed in a given time
- information on any follow-up or concurrent necessary treatment
- advice and product information to be given to the patient and/or carer, including side effects, interactions, contra-indications, precautions etc. (including the use of manufacturers' product information leaflets)

Continued

Nurse		
Designation		
Competency/qualifications	Indicators	Assessed

(*continued*) identification and management of adverse events or outcomes; the concurrent use of other drugs/medicines)

- arrangements for referral to a doctor when desired or necessary
- facilities and supplies which should be readily available

Training

Pharmacy course prior to use of protocol – content as agreed by the Patient Services Committee (Mallett *et al.* 1998)	Successful completion of course as assessed by agreed clinical assessor and nurse	
Yearly update training by pharmacy		
Review of competency	One year following last competency assessment as assessed by the nurse, and the hospital agreed assessor	

Index